CONTENTS

FOREWORD

Having been involved in the world of voice-hearing since I heard my first voice in 1982, I quickly found myself trapped in a psychiatric system that was determined to treat me as ill. Even my protestations of wellness were viewed in this world as part of my illness. For ten years I remained an impatient patient, labelled a 'treatment-resistant schizophrenic'. I spent most of my day in bed and, during the hours I was awake, was in a near comatose state induced either by my treatment (medication) or copious amounts of alcohol (my medication of choice). Ten years into my psychiatric career I became involved in a fledgling organisation called the Hearing Voices Network.

In this Network I slowly became aware of a different way of viewing voices. In the first instance it was the group of voice-hearers that met in Manchester, England who explained to me that it was possible to live with voices – even those that were distressing. Secondly, it was a man named Terry McLaughlin who not only befriended me but also showed me I could move beyond coping with my voices into a stage of living with my voices. The third factor for me in these early days was the work of Marius Romme and Sandra Escher, both of whom remain close friends and mentors. They showed me that not only could I live with my voices, but that I could work through my experience and take control of my voices.

All of the above encouraged me to read as much as I could about voices. This led me to the present work. When I first read *Hearing Voices: A Common Human Experience* I once again felt my stance on voice-hearing was vindicated and knew immediately that here was someone who, like Romme and Escher, really understood something of the voice-hearers' experience. Having read the book on its first print run I found it to be one of the most sensitively thought through pieces of writing that explored the issue of voice-hearing. The first time I met John I knew why: John Watkins is a man of real intellect and sensitivity, two qualities rarely found together. This book will, I am sure, affect many people in a positive way. When it was first published it was a book ahead of its time. Now, readers will find in these pages a book whose time has come.

Ron Coleman

INTRODUCTION

Inner voices, invisible companions, the voice of conscience, locutions, inner guides, spirits, angels, demons, ghosts, muses, thoughts-out-loud, radio waves of divinity, the voice of God, language magic, the Other Order, cold castigation language, persecutors, court-of-law punishment language, self-talk, inner helpers, splinter psyches, sub-personalities, auditory hallucinations. These and many other terms have been used to refer to voices which have no ordinary physical cause. The very diversity of these names reflects the enormous variety of experiences that human beings can have, which can range from the sublime and spiritually uplifting 'locutions' described by many saints and mystics, through to seemingly malevolent invisible 'presences' which verbally harass, threaten and attack.

If the various kinds of voice hearing experiences have anything in common it is that they are poorly understood and often harshly judged. By encouraging readers to think about voices in a new way I hope this book will lead to greater understanding of these experiences and more helpful attitudes toward those who have them. I feel that it is important to state at the outset that the book evolved out of my long-standing interest in schizophrenia, a psychological disturbance with which hearing voices is often associated. A feeling of restless discontent with what I saw as a lack of depth in the conventional approaches to helping people with this and other mental disorders drove me to seek alternative ways of understanding the often inexplicable experiences of my clients. My research, which at first simply involved a closer examination of the actual experiences of persons living with schizophrenia, soon led to the realisation that the little I knew about hearing voices was merely

1

the 'tip of the iceberg', beneath which lay an expansive, uncharted and seldom explored realm. This realisation, which would alone have justified the considerable effort I expended, turned out to be only the beginning of an eye-opening journey of discovery. My initial feeling of being driven gradually turned into one of being drawn as, with mounting curiosity and fascination, my awareness opened onto much broader vistas than I could have imagined. I was eventually led to an appreciation of the fact that, in whatever form it occurs, hearing voices is a phenomenon of great significance, both practical and theoretical, for a vast range of individuals, social and cultural groups, and humankind as a whole.

The book begins with a description of voice experiences themselves, and firstly with those that occur among members of the general population. No doubt many readers will be surprised to learn how prevalent voice hearing is among human beings commonly referred to as 'normal'! In subsequent chapters spiritual voice experiences and those associated with various types of mental disorder are described. In all of these accounts I have endeavoured to remain as close as possible to actual experiences people have described. Readers primarily interested in learning about the formal characteristics of different kinds of voice experiences can take the descriptions provided in the first few chapters as a reliable introduction to the phenomenon since they mainly consist of first-hand reports. It is very important to remember that such reports are really all we have to go on when it comes to learning about the actual human *experience* of hearing voices since, even in this era of enthrallment with 'high tech' approaches, there is no electronic apparatus or other device which can provide any insight whatever into what is occurring in the hearer's *mind*, whatever it might reveal about what their brain is doing!

Readers will discover that voice hearing occurs under very many different circumstances and takes a bewildering variety of forms, ranging from the relatively common experience in which a person hears their name called out loud while falling asleep through to the extraordinarily moving encounters related by those who have had profound spiritual experiences. As will be seen, not only can voice experiences with distinctly spiritual qualities deeply affect the person who has them, they may also have reverberations which go well beyond the individual to affect the values and beliefs of large groups of people, possibly even entire societies.

Chapter One

HEARING VOICES:
A COMMON HUMAN EXPERIENCE

*Voices have spoken to our predecessors throughout human
history. They can speak to us today, if we will listen, and if
we apply the discernment and understanding that is also
available to us in this modern era.*

– Mitchell Liester[1]

The experience of hearing voices speaking 'when there is no one
there' is often considered to be one of the classic hallmarks of
severe mental disorder. Those who hold such views may be rather
surprised, therefore, to discover just how common such experiences
actually are. Over at least the past one hundred years surveys of
fully awake, healthy, 'normal' adults have consistently revealed that
very many people have heard one or more disembodied voices
speaking to them at some time during their lives. Indeed, it appears
that a *majority* of ordinary, well-adjusted people have had such
experiences at least once, and a significant number of others have
had them more often.

There is enormous individual variability both in the kinds of
voice experiences human beings are capable of having and in their
responses and reactions to them. For example, some experiences
are very brief – they may only last for a few seconds – and never
occur again. On the other hand, some voices continue over a much
longer time, perhaps even for many years. The subjective impact
of voices on the hearer also covers a wide spectrum of
possibilities. Some are comforting and helpful, perhaps even
inspiring, and enrich the hearer's life considerably. On the other
hand, however, there are many people who are tormented by
harshly critical or commanding voices which they feel powerless
to escape from or control.

The Occurrence of Voices in the Human Population

Despite the fact that voice experiences are quite common their actual prevalence is very difficult to determine with any real accuracy. This is partly because of the fear and stigma which surrounds a phenomenon which many people in Western societies are still inclined to automatically associate with 'madness'. In an effort to avoid the shame and embarrassment of being derogatively accused of 'hearing things' many people understandably choose not to disclose to others what they have actually experienced. In spite of these and various other difficulties a substantial body of evidence has been gathered regarding this fascinating aspect of human psychology. In some of the studies discussed below care was taken to protect the anonymity of those participating in interviews or completing questionnaires, which thereby encouraged them to respond more truthfully than they may otherwise have felt comfortable doing. The results of this research are often surprising.

The most extensive survey of voice hearing experiences to date was carried out in England, Russia and Brazil in the early 1890s by Professor Henry Sidgwick and his colleagues on behalf of the newly-formed Society for Psychical Research under the auspices of the International Congress of Experimental Psychology.[2] Although the selection of subjects for this 'International Census of Waking Hallucinations in the Sane' was not random persons who had any obvious physical illness or mental disorder were excluded from participation. Survey respondents were asked to answer the following single question:

> Have you ever, when believing yourself to be completely awake, had a vivid impression of seeing or being touched by a living being or inanimate object, or of hearing a voice; which impression, as far as you could discover, was not due to any external physical cause?

Responses were obtained from a total of 17,000 persons of whom 1,684 (9.9%) answered in the affirmative. A total of 493 (approximately 2.9% of the total group) reported having had the experience of hearing a voice. Interestingly, voice experiences having some kind of religious or supernatural content represented a small but significant minority of these reports, some of which were claimed to be veridical (i.e. to correspond to an actual external event).

During the course of the century following Professor Sidgwick's pioneering investigation the findings of many other researchers have been consistently similar.[3] One recent study focused specifically on the experience of hearing voices among 375 mentally healthy college students. The researchers who administered the survey repeatedly emphasised the fact that 'hearing voices' meant hearing a voice fully aloud 'as if someone had spoken'. The results revealed that 71% of the students had had some kind of experience with voices whilst fully awake. Five general types of voice experiences were identified in this study: hearing a voice calling one's name aloud when alone (reported by 36% of the students); hearing one's thoughts as if spoken aloud (39%); hearing one's name when falling asleep (30%); hearing a comforting or advising voice (10%); and hearing God's voice (11%). Approximately 5% of the students also reported having held a conversation with a voice (which was usually that of some familiar person such as a dead grandmother, absent friend, or mother). The psychologists who conducted this research concluded that hearing voices is a rather common experience although it is seldom reported or discussed. Indeed, their findings suggested that the experience of hearing voices may occur at one time or another in a *majority* of the 'normal' human population:

> The results of this study demonstrate that brief and occasional auditory hallucinations [i.e. voices] of particular types are reasonably common among the college student population. Indeed, the results suggest that perhaps more than half of the normal population may have some experience with voice hallucinations, particularly those of hearing one's name called, and/or hearing one's thoughts aloud ... If our results are reliable, one would wonder why such common experiences are widely believed to be so uncommon.[4]

The 'inner voice' experiences of 30 people were studied by Myrtle Heery in 1989.[5] Half the subjects in this study were known to the author whilst the other 15 were randomly selected from 50 questionnaire respondents. A range of experiences were described by these people, many of them involving personal growth or spiritual issues. The author noted that her subjects had a wide range of occupations and incomes, with 93% possessing a college education or a higher degree. Commenting on the widely held view that the experience of hearing voices is exclusively linked with sainthood or psychosis, Heery concluded that ordinary men and women who are 'neither saints nor psychotics' also often hear inner voices.

In recent years others who have studied voice hearing experiences have reached similar conclusions. Thus, nearly a century after Professor Sidgwick's original survey, a 1991 analysis of data provided by the US National Institute of Mental Health on 15,000 members of the general population revealed that 2.3% had experienced 'auditory hallucinations' of some kind whilst fully awake.[6] These experiences were most common in 18–19 year olds with a second peak in 40–49 year olds and a further rise after about age 65 or 70. Interestingly, only about one in three persons had told a professional about their experience or felt that it caused distress or impaired their ability to function.

The results of a carefully controlled study in 1992 involving 586 college students led the psychologist researchers to conclude that a relatively large majority of people in the general population have frequent voice experiences and that these are not related to any kind of mental disorder.[7] Participants in this particular study reported experiences such as hearing their own name spoken out loud in a store (64.0%) or when in a house alone (32.8%); hearing their own thoughts spoken out loud (37.2%); hearing their own name when falling asleep (24.6%); hearing the voice of an absent friend (11%) or dead relative (6%); and hearing God's voice (8.7%). Whilst many of the students (23%) stated that the experience had only occurred once or twice ever, 45% said that it occurred between once a day and once a month. These findings suggested to the researchers that 'a relatively common phenomenon in normal consciousness may have been entirely overlooked'. Julian Jaynes, a Princeton University psychology professor and prominent researcher on voice experiences, has commented on the implications of such findings as follows:

> Auditory verbal hallucinations [i.e. voices] exist in varying percentages in every population in the world where they have been studied. They are of course most notable nowadays in severely stressed individuals that we label schizophrenic. But, contrary to what many an ardent

biological psychiatrist wishes to think, they occur in normal individuals also, and they are not always indicative of pathology. This has been known for over a century.[8]

The Observations of Early Psychologists

In 1832 the French physician Jean Esquirol defined the concept of hallucination that is still widely used today. In his influential monograph, *Mental Maladies: A Treatise on Insanity*, Esquirol noted that various kinds of hallucinatory experiences were extremely common among persons considered to be mentally disturbed. He went on to note, however, that hallucinatory experiences – including those which involve hearing voices – may also occur in persons who are normal or even superior in their mental functioning:

> If hallucinations are most frequently the lot of feeble minds, men the most remarkable for their strength of understanding, the depth of their reason, and their vigour of thought, are not always free from this symptom.[9]

In 1883 one of the greatest of the early pioneers of psychology, Francis Galton, published his treatise entitled *Inquiries Into Human Faculty and Its Development*. During the preparation of this work Galton's attention was drawn to an unexpected phenomenon which led him to state: 'The number of sane persons who see visions . . . is much greater than I had any idea of when I began this study.' Furthermore, the many first-hand accounts Galton was able to collect soon showed him that these experiences were not confined to the visual sphere:

> A notable proportion of sane persons have had not only visions, but actual hallucinations of sight, sound, or other sense, at one or more periods of their lives. I have a considerable packet of instances contributed by my personal friends, besides a large number communicated to me by other correspondents. . . . [One] lady, apparently in vigorous health, and belonging to a vigorous family, told me that during some past months she had been plagued by voices. The words were at first simple nonsense; then the word 'pray' was frequently repeated; this was followed by

some more or less coherent sentences of little import, and finally the voices left her. In short, the familiar hallucinations of the insane are to be met with far more frequently than is commonly supposed, among people moving in society and in good working health.[10]

In addition to the unexpectedly high prevalence of hallucinatory experiences in the general population, Galton was impressed by the frequency with which 'great men' have been subject to these phenomena. As an example he cited the case of Socrates (see below), 'whose daimon was an audible not a visual appearance'.

The eminent psychologist and philosopher William James, who is often regarded as the founder of modern psychology, was the American agent for Professor Sidgwick's 'Census of Hallucinations'. James did not believe that hearing voices was necessarily a pathological phenomenon, and in 1892 he stated so in his influential textbook of psychology:

> Most of the 'voices' which people hear ... are described as 'inner voices', although their character is entirely unlike the inner speech of the subject with himself. I know of several people who hear such inner voices making unforeseen remarks whenever they grow quiet and listen for them. They are a very common incident of delusional insanity, and may at last grow into vivid or completely exteriorised hallucinations. The latter are comparatively frequent occurrences in sporadic form; and certain individuals are liable to have them often. From the results of the 'Census of Hallucinations' ... it would appear that, roughly speaking, one person at least in every ten is likely to have had a vivid hallucination at some time in his life.[11]

James noted that the most common hallucination of all was the experience of hearing one's own name called aloud: nearly half of the 'sporadic cases' he collected were of this kind.

Specific Circumstances in Which Voices May Be Heard

In addition to those which seem to just come from 'out of the blue' there are a very wide range of circumstances in which mentally healthy individuals may have voice experiences of one kind or another. The following are among the most common of them:

1 *Hypnagogic and Hypnopompic Experiences*

A wide range of experiences involving vivid imagery often occur during the period intermediate between wakefulness and sleep. The term 'hypnagogic' refers to imagery associated with the onset of sleep, whilst 'hypnopompic' refers to imagery which occurs as a person is waking up. These *normal* hallucination-like phenomena sometimes involve hearing sounds with great clarity and intensity. In several studies more than 70% of adults reported having had hypnagogic experiences, whilst hypnopompic experiences appear somewhat less common. Hypnagogic experiences often involve hearing sounds, music or voices. Hearing one's name called is especially common and is sometimes so vivid that people have been known to arise from their bed in order to investigate its source. Whilst they are waking from sleep some people describe hearing a familiar voice (such as their mother or a room-mate) encouraging them to wake up. The specific content of hypnagogic voices often seems nonsensical or bizarre:

> Often the sounds are meaningless, or so they seem. Sometimes they are neologisms, e.g. 'Lacertina Wein', 'they are exposed to verbally intellection', 'or squawms of medication allowed me to ungather', 'anzeema', or strange remarks apparently heard in one's own voice such as 'I wanted to pull seven but I pulled nine instead', irrelevant sentences containing unrecognisable names like 'Bill Hambra – Ju know him', pompous nonsense often characterised by unintellectual wit, e.g. 'Buy stocks in the fixed stars. It is remarkably stable', 'he is as good as cake double', 'a leading clerk is a great thing in my profession, as well as a Sabine footertootro'.[12]

On the other hand, hypnagogic voices sometimes seem to be meaningfully related to the person's current thoughts. For example, one person who was attempting to closely examine these phenomena had the following experience:

> I was trying to pick up hypnagogic experiences and heard,

'Still a nothing.' I wasn't getting much and it said as much. While I was trying to see in detail how the hypnagogic experience forms I heard, 'Do you have a computer?' I was getting very sleepy in the hypnagogic state and heard, 'The usual snoofing.' At the time the odd word 'snoofing' sounded like a cross between snooping (trying to snoop on the hypnagogic) and snoozing (getting sleepy). It was a playful representation of where I was – both snooping and snoozing.[13]

Many cases have been reported in which people on the brink of sleep have heard the voice of a friend or loved one who conveyed significant information to them.[14] In some instances such voices were recognised to belong to someone who was later found to have died at the very same moment their voice was heard.[15] (A discussion of voice experiences and paranormal phenomena can be found in Chapter Six.)

2 *Dreams*

Dreams are sometimes described as hallucinations which occur during sleep. Like hypnagogic and hypnopompic experiences, they can be considered a common type of *normal* hallucination.[16] The similarity between dream experiences and the hallucinatory voices of psychosis has long been recognised. Thus, in his classic monograph on schizophrenia, Professor Eugen Bleuler noted that 'The human dream-life is identical with the sphere of the voices of the insane.'[17] Whilst dreams are often primarily visual the auditory aspects sometimes constitute their most compelling sensory feature. In fact, some people have dreams which are predominantly auditory. The voices heard in dreams may belong to the dreamer or to a person or persons known or unknown to them. In some dreams the voices are ascribed to non-human sources such as inanimate objects, animals or supernatural beings. The early Egyptians and Greeks developed the art of 'incubation' or 'temple sleep' in order to facilitate the experience of revelatory dreams. The belief that significant verbal messages may be conveyed in dreams continues in many contemporary cultures. As an example, Moroccan Jews on pilgrimage in Israel highly value 'visitational dreams' in which they may see a revered saint who speaks to them and answers their questions in an experience which is felt to have profound healing potential.[18] (The relationship between voices and dreams is considered further in Chapter Six.)

3 *Imaginary Companions of Childhood*

It is common for children to have an imaginary companion for at least some period whilst they are growing up. Such imaginary companions are especially prevalent during the preschool years and usually take the form of a playmate. In one study of 141 three and four-year olds, 65% reported having such playmates.[19] In most cases these companions disappear after a year or two, though sometimes they persist into adolescence and possibly even into adulthood. In many instances children are able to actually hear the voice of their imaginary playmate:

> Those who have studied the phenomena of 'imaginary playmates' (which should read hallucinated playmates) are convinced that such children hear the 'voices' of their (by us unseen) friends in their conversations with them. In my own studies, I have found that about half the women students at a religious college had had hallucinated playmates, half of these clearly remembering the pitch and quality of the voices. One of these women still has her hallucinated playmates, now grown up like her, who appear in times of stress, their voices clearly 'heard' and not imagined. She is not psychotic.[20]

Among the 375 college students in the study referred to earlier, 25% said they had had an imaginary companion in childhood and 6% said they heard the playmate's voice aloud and it was 'just like a real voice'.

4 *Bereavement and Mourning*

Grief and mourning are a part of the normal process of bereavement which follows the loss of a loved one. Research has revealed that during bereavement it is very common for people to see, hear or feel the presence of the deceased person. Recently bereaved elderly people, in particular, very frequently report having such experiences which in some cases continue for many years. For example, in a

recent study of 50 bereaved people in their early seventies, 82%
reported having felt the presence of the deceased person and many
also said they spoke to, heard or saw them during the first month
of bereavement (89% of those describing such experiences were
women and 57% men).[21] At least 30% of these people told of having
heard the voice of the deceased person during this time. The
following experience is a simple example of this phenomenon:

> One interviewed subject recounted hearing her grand-
> father's voice from next to her ear shortly after learning
> that he had died. She described standing in her closet
> selecting a dress to pack for the funeral when the voice said
> 'Wear that one, I've always liked it'.[22]

When interviewed again after 12 months had elapsed, 52% of the
subjects were still having these experiences (54% of the women and
46% of the men). In one group of 293 widows and widowers, 52.6%
still reported having these experiences 10 years after their spouse
died, and after 20 years 42.7% said they still had them. Forty years
afterwards 31.8% were still having some kind of sensory experience
involving their loved one.[23] These 'bereavement hallucinations'
seem to be especially common among people who have had a long
and happy marriage. Interestingly, the surviving spouses of unhappy
marriages seem unlikely to have them! Significantly, they are *not*
associated with depression or any other kind of psychological or
physical abnormality. In fact, the experience of hearing the voice
of a deceased spouse is considered to be pleasant and helpful by
the majority of widows and widowers. In some instances it is taken
to be tangible evidence of the survival of the 'spirit' of the deceased
person following their bodily demise.

Children and adolescents may also hear a voice during the acute
grief reaction following the death of a parent. Often this experience
involves the child hearing the dead parent giving admonitions and
prohibitions to them.[24] The experience of hearing or seeing a
recently deceased family member is especially common in certain
ethnic groups (e.g. among the Hopi Indians of North America).[25]
The 'hallucinations' which are common among elderly nursing
home residents sometimes involve the experience of sensory contact
with the deceased – although they may not necessarily be
recognised as such.[26]

Although the voices heard by the bereaved are often confined to a few words or to short, simple sentences this is not always the case. Longer and more complex interactions have also been reported, as was the case for a woman who, almost every morning, had long, informative, and pleasant conversations with the voice of her dead grandmother in which the grandmother's voice was actually heard.[27] In some instances the bereaved person is also able to see a visual image of the deceased and a two-way conversation takes place between them. The communication which results may sometimes have profound consequences for the bereaved individual as the following anecdote clearly shows:

> My granddad died of a massive heart attack whilst Gran was out playing lawn bowls. He'd been a difficult man, but their marriage had lasted for around sixty years. They'd shared a broad interest in spiritual matters and, although an intensely practical woman, Gran believed in the possibility of communication with the deceased. Some two weeks after Grandad's death I was staying with her. She'd aged ten or more years in those two weeks and the family were all concerned she wouldn't be far behind Grandad. She said she could no longer play bowls because she felt so guilty at having been there, enjoying herself, when he died. Bowls had sustained her and given her great pleasure over more years than I could recall. One evening, with a strong sense of urgency, Gran told me that she would not be able to go on if she couldn't communicate with Grandad. She needed some indication from him that it was alright for her to continue on and enjoy her life. She was also surprised that they had not already communicated by this stage and saw it as an ominous sign. The morning after this conversation Gran appeared from her room a changed woman. Her greyish-looking skin had regained its usual brown colour and there was a lightness about her. Her spirit appeared to have returned: she and Grandad had communicated. Although we never discussed the contents of their communication it was obvious to all of us that this experience had changed her life. She went on to live another sixteen years as the feisty, strong-willed woman she had always been.[28]

Despite the fact that these kinds of experiences are a normal and often helpful aspect of bereavement most people who have them do not disclose them to anyone – not even to relatives, close friends, clergy, or medical personnel – for fear of possible negative reactions such as being judged mentally abnormal. By contrast, in cultures such as Japan where no stigma is associated with such experiences bereaved persons who have them do not needlessly become fearful about their sanity.[29] In fact, in many non-Western societies it is taken for granted that these kinds of experiences are related to contact with the 'spirit' of the deceased person.[30] Some authorities have recommended that, since such experiences may be *expected* to occur in the newly bereaved, both the bereaved person and others concerned should be counselled to accept them as normal in order to alleviate fear and prevent unnecessary worry and other negative reactions.

5 *Severe Stress, Anxiety and Trauma*

A wide range of hallucinatory phenomena may occur in association with stressors such as sleep deprivation, profound isolation, serious illness, solitary confinement, torture, hunger, thirst, sensory deprivation, and bereavement.[31] It appears that stress of sufficient severity can act as a 'trigger' which will instigate the experience of hearing voices in certain individuals. Persistent auditory hallucinations in the form of voices have been found to occur in a significant number of persons who have developed a post-traumatic stress disorder (PTSD).[32] Some people who have been subjected to continuing high levels of stress have described hearing the comforting voice of a parent or other significant and reassuring person, as in the following example:

> I had rather an emotional crisis some years ago . . . I felt a presence somehow, in my bedroom, and I thought it was my old grandmother who'd been dead for some years. I could have sworn I saw her there and I spoke to her in Welsh. She said, 'You are in trouble my son and I may be able to help you.'[33]

Similar 'benign hallucinations' sometimes occur when a person is undergoing the stress of hospitalisation for medical or surgical reasons, as in this example:

A man, recovering after an acute coronary thrombosis, heard a 'voice' say: 'You are saved.' Being of religious inclination, he attributed it to the many prayers he had offered up for his deliverance.[34]

The profound trauma of childhood sexual abuse appears to be a common precursor of voice experiences. In one recent study it was found that 27% of incest victims heard voices later in their lives.[35] Indeed, there is growing evidence that the extreme distress associated with prolonged childhood physical, emotional or sexual abuse may be a major factor in the development of voices which take the form of imaginary companions or the 'alter' personalities of multiple personality disorder (MPD).[36] (PTSD and MPD are discussed in detail in later chapters.)

6 Extreme Deprivation and Isolation

People deprived of food, water or sleep for extended periods often become prone to experiencing hallucinations of various kinds.[37] In sensory deprivation experiments subjects who are exposed to conditions of minimal visual, auditory and tactile stimulation by being placed in a darkened and sound-proofed room for days at a time have reported experiencing vivid sensory imagery which sometimes reaches hallucinatory proportions.[38] Certain kinds of illness or injury that require treatment which exposes the patient to a significantly reduced level of sensory and social stimulation have occasionally been found to facilitate the development of psychotic episodes which are accompanied by hallucinatory experiences. For example, severely burned patients who are totally immobilised and covered with bandages (including their eyes) have been known to experience psychotic episodes.[39] In recent years it has been recognised that states of relative sensory deprivation ('sensory poverty') such as may be experienced by patients faced with prolonged isolation and immobilisation in post-operative recovery rooms and intensive care units, may also contribute significantly to the development of post-operative psychosis and delirium:

> Sensory deprivation is now frequently recognised as an important feature in the care of some patients with transient psychotic states or sensory deprivation symptoms, especially in hospitalised patients and in those with severe

handicaps, such as blindness, deafness, and paralysis ... The well-meaning physician's hospital orders may turn out to be a sentence of sensory deprivation, with excessive or too long-enduring absolute bed rest, silence, and no visitors. The patient may be found wandering in the corridors – usually at night when the wards have become quiet – confused, thinking he is at home, and being unable to find a familiar room. Sensory deprivation has loosened his hold on reality and has made him prey to fantasy.[40]

Circumstances involving extreme and prolonged social isolation may provoke unusual experiences similar to those which occur in sensory deprivation experiments. Individuals who are confined to constricted or remote situations, either alone or in small groups, may be subject to the effects of both social and (relative) sensory deprivation. Solo aviators, polar explorers, mountain climbers, astronauts, lone sailors, submarine crews, and radar watch-keepers, among others, have all reported various unusual perceptual experiences associated with their isolated circumstances. Persons undergoing prolonged involuntary social isolation, such as lost explorers, prisoners in solitary confinement, and shipwrecked sailors, have also described having a range of hallucinatory experiences during their lonely and stressful ordeals.[41] For example, Charles Lindbergh, the first man to fly solo across the Atlantic, has described 'phantom figures' that spoke to him with familiar human voices during his pioneering journey:

> While I'm staring at the instruments, during an unearthly age of time, both conscious and asleep, the fuselage behind me becomes filled with ghostly presences – vaguely outlined forms, transparent, moving, riding weightless with me in the plane. I feel no surprise at their coming ... Without turning my head, I see them as clearly as though in my normal field of vision ... These phantoms speak with human voices ... First one and then another presses forward to my shoulder to speak above the engine's noise, and then draws back among the group behind. At times, voices come out of the air itself, clear yet far away, travelling through distances that can't be measured by the scale of human miles; familiar voices, conversing and advising on my flight, discussing problems of my

navigation, reassuring me, giving me messages of importance unattainable in ordinary life.[42]

It is not known how common these kinds of experiences may be among persons who, as a result of profound physical illness or disability, are cut off from normal levels of social, emotional, and intellectual stimulation.* A recent study of a group of cerebral palsied, spastic-athetoid, quadriplegic adults, all of whom were totally dependent on others and unable to speak, has raised the possibility that they may actually be quite common. When a system of communicating with these persons was developed it was discovered that many seemed to be hearing voices. Usually the voices were felt to be helpful, for example encouraging participation in training programmes. The researchers concluded that, for certain physically handicapped populations, such experiences 'may be the rule, not the exception'.[43]

A significant reduction in auditory acuity (deafness) may contribute to the experience of auditory hallucinations, especially in the elderly. Thus, people with a long history of progressive bilateral hearing loss sometimes describe hearing instrumental music, singing, and voices.[44] Hallucinations associated with sensory deficits have been referred to as 'release hallucinations' since they often involve memory traces of earlier experiences being released into awareness as a consequence of the low level of external sensory input.[45] It is possible that such experiences may occur as a consequence of the state of chronic sensory deprivation which sometimes accompanies profound deafness.

In some cultural contexts people actively seek or create situations of extreme sensory and social deprivation in order to facilitate the emergence of hallucinatory experiences which they believe have a religious or spiritual significance. In ancient Greece, for example, persons seeking oracular revelations from the god Trophonius would descend into the darkened caverns at Lebadea, sometimes remaining there alone for days at a time.[46] Islamic

---

* The fact that hallucinations of various kinds may be elicited in *many* people under conditions of extreme social isolation raises the possibility that people with a psychotic disorder such as schizophrenia who have become largely cut off from the normal social world might experience hallucinatory voices as a result of their sensory isolation alone.

tradition maintains that the angel Gabriel appeared and dictated the Koran to Mohammed whilst he was meditating alone in the cave of Hira. According to the New Testament it was during the forty days of his lonely sojourn in the wilderness that the devil appeared and spoke to Jesus and tempted him. (Spiritual aspects of voice experiences are discussed in detail in the next chapter.)

7 Hypnotic Experiences

Vivid experiences involving hearing voices can often be induced in hypnotised subjects by means of suggestion.[47] An illustration of this is provided by the following experiment in which a realistic two-way conversation took place between a hypnotised subject (in this instance, the philosopher Aldous Huxley) and the subject's 'wife' who 'appeared' to him following covert suggestions made by the hypnotherapist Milton Erickson:

> [Huxley] expressed surprise at his wife's unexpected return since he had expected her to be absent the entire day . . . He conversed with her and apparently hallucinated replies. He was interrupted with the question of how he knew that it was his wife and not an hypnotic hallucination. He examined the question thoughtfully, then explained that I had not given him any suggestion to hallucinate his wife [hence] it was reasonable to assume that she was a reality. After a brief thoughtful pause, he returned to his 'conversation' with her apparently continuing to hallucinate replies. Finally I attracted his attention and made a hand gesture suggestive of a disappearance toward the chair in which he 'saw' his wife. To his complete astonishment he saw her slowly fade away.[48]

It has been suggested by some authorities that in certain cases people who hear persistent voices may actually be unknowingly generating the voices themselves by means of a form of spontaneous 'self-hypnosis'.[49] (This possibility is discussed further in Chapter Six.)

8 *Near Death Experiences*

Whether medically-induced or spontaneous the recovery of people who have been close to death (in some cases involving actual clinical death) has led to the recognition that many such persons undergo intense and profoundly moving experiences whilst in the near-death state.[50] According to one recent study more than 40% of people who have survived near-death crises report having had such experiences.[51] It has been estimated that as many as 8 million Americans may have had a near-death experience.[52] Descriptions collected from a wide range of autobiographical accounts have established that the near-death experience (NDE) is typically characterised by a number of the following: feelings of peace; an out-of-body experience; the sensation of travelling very quickly through a dark tunnel, usually towards a brilliant light; an encounter with the spirits of deceased relatives or friends or a 'Being of Light'; an instantaneous life review and, in some cases, final entry into a 'world of light'.

Whilst travelling towards 'the Light' many people describe being stopped or turned back following an encounter with the presence of a spiritual being of some kind. This spiritual presence often takes the form of a voice which instructs the person to 'go back'. The following experience related by a forty-four year old man who attempted suicide whilst deeply depressed is a typical example of this kind of experience:

> I was trying to get to a distant light that I could see. It was a brilliant light of some sort, and I wanted to get to it but I could feel this tug, tugging me back. And then I distinctly remember a voice saying, 'Well, Robert, you're not finished yet – you have to go back. You're not ready, you're not finished with what you have to do.' That was the impression I got, those sort of words. I tried my hardest to pull towards the brilliant light [but] after I heard the voice, I can remember coming back, and as I was coming back I could even sort of feel myself coming down towards my body. And then I remember waking up in the Intensive Care Unit some time later. I must admit after it happened I thought perhaps it might have been the depression that had something to do with the vision, but then I felt it

couldn't have been that because it felt so vivid and so good.[53]

People who have had near-death experiences often feel that the voice told them that they had to decide for themselves what they wanted to do. A twenty-five year old woman whose NDE occurred whilst she was giving birth to her first child had the following voice experience:

> There was light at the end of the tunnel and it was glowing. It was very welcoming and warm and I wanted to get there. I was more concerned about getting there than staying where I was. I almost reached the light, but then I stopped. I looked back and it was as though I was very high above the hospital ... Then I heard a voice saying very clearly, 'What do you want to do?' I was given the choice, but I knew I had to go back. I knew I'd only been asked the question because I had to go back, I was needed. And I said, 'I have to go back.' And the voice said, 'Yes.' And I went back down and came back into myself again.[54]

Some people continue to hear the voice long after their complete physical recovery. An example of this is provided by a woman who, eighteen months after a NDE, was still seeking to find her purpose in life. She had begun to have serious doubts about her earlier experience but quite unexpectedly one day everything changed:

> I was standing there cooking, stirring a sauce, and being fairly introspective, and thinking, 'What is it, God, that you want me to do?' At this point I just heard the same inner voice that I'd been confronted with when I left my body during the NDE. That presence of love came back and said, 'Pick up a pen and write down what you hear.' I thought I was going crazy, but after the third time of hearing it – 'Pick up the pen and write down what you hear' – I did it. And I started to ask questions: 'What is it we are to do?' I was told that same afternoon that we were to go to the mountains in the south to make a place of rest and solace for many in the future. After that it was incredible – every time I wanted to ask something, there was the answer. I knew it was coming from something external to myself, but

within myself, if you can understand. I had answers of a spiritual depth that I knew wasn't me.[55]

People attribute the voice they hear during a NDE to a range of different possible sources. For example, some people feel it belonged to someone they know, such as a relative or dear friend. Some medical patients at first thought it was their doctor's voice but discovered later that it was not. Some feel certain that the voice belonged to a spiritual or divine entity, such as God, an angel, or 'the Light' itself.

9 Psychedelic Experiences

A multitude of chemical substances, both naturally occurring and synthetic, are known to induce altered states of consciousness (ASCs) in which hallucinatory experiences of various kinds often occur.[56] Drugs such as LSD, psilocybine ('magic mushrooms'), mescaline ('peyote') and a number of others are referred to as 'psychedelic', which is often interpreted to mean 'mind-expanding', although the alternative term 'hallucinogenic' is sometimes used in order to emphasise their potential to induce hallucinations. Although the sensory experiences associated with psychedelic ASCs are often predominantly visual in nature auditory hallucinations of sounds, music or voices can also occur. The following experience occurred during an LSD-induced 'trip':

> I had several hallucinations that I recognised as such. At one point elves appeared and accepted me as a jolly fellow spirit. They spoke to me in verse and wanted to guide me to magical places – to castles and mythological realms. Many different personalities, all of them part of oneself, became autonomous and spoke of various things.[57]

In many traditional cultures naturally-occurring psychedelic substances are used in the context of shamanic practices in order to facilitate contact with what is believed to be the 'spirit world'. Such experiences may involve the subject being spoken to and guided by 'spirits'. In some instances initiation into the role of shaman follows the receipt of a 'call' from the spirit world. This phenomenon is illustrated by the following experience associated with the ritual ingestion of 'magic mushrooms':

I had to eat the mushrooms three times and the man from San Lucas, who gave them to me, proposed his work as a medicine man to me, telling me: now you are going to receive my study. I asked him why he thought I was going to receive it when I didn't want to learn anything about his wisdom, I only wanted to get better and be cured of my illness. Then he answered me: now it is no longer you who command . . . Then I heard the voice of my father. He had been dead for forty-three years when he spoke to me the first time I ate the mushrooms: This work that is being given to you, he said, I am he who tells you to accept it . . . I couldn't imagine from where this voice came that was speaking to me. Then it was that the shaman of San Lucas told me that the voice I was hearing was that of my father.[58]

Shamanic initiation experiences such as this conform to the original meaning of the term 'vocation', i.e. to be called by an inner voice (see below). (Shamanism is discussed in detail in the next chapter.)

10 *Creative Inspiration*

The 'Muses' that are often credited with inspiring the creativity of poets and musicians sometimes assume a tangible sensory form. A significant number of individuals who have produced highly regarded artistic works claim to have been inspired or guided by voices. Writers, in particular, have sometimes been quite adamant that the 'true' authors of their creations were invisible presences that spoke directly to them and that their own role was merely to serve as a faithful amanuensis. The acclaimed German poet Rilke, for example, is said to have taken down a long sonnet sequence that he heard spoken to him by a voice and John Milton alluded to his 'Celestial Patroness, who . . . unimplor'd . . . dictates to me my unpremeditated Verse'.[59] The visionary artist and poet William Blake (1757–1827), who held animated conversations with the long-dead Milton, insisted that many of his own works were created under the direction of 'Messengers from Heaven' and that much of his poetry was 'dictated' to him by 'celestial friends' whilst he merely acted as a 'secretary' taking down this dictation.[60]

Inner voices played a major role in the creative life of one of the greatest of the Romantic composers, Robert Schumann (1810–1856). As well as helping him to finally decide on a career as a composer the voices helped him produce some of his most important musical compositions. Schumann personified two of his voices and gave them the names 'Florestan' and 'Eusebius':

> 'Florestan' ... over the years became the confident, extrovert and manly alter ego. Schumann liked to see 'Florestan the Improviser' as his 'bosom friend ... my own ego'. The other voice that haunted him came slightly later, and was to be christened 'Eusebius'. This was Schumann's more sensitive, withdrawn, passive, feminine part ... once they appeared, the solitary Schumann was often to be found talking to his selves ... Above all, the sounds he heard in his head led him to compose at the piano. He often wrote music under 'dictation': 'gods were coming out of my fingers'. At a later, mature stage in his career, he believed his inner voices dictated to him his Spring Symphony and his Manfred Overture. These noises ... helped guide him towards, and convince him of, his true vocation: being a composer.[61]

Like William Blake, Schumann felt that some of his most significant musical compositions were made under 'dictation' from the voices he heard. It was 'Florestan' and 'Eusebius', he said, who dictated to him his *Spring Symphony* and his *Manfred Overture*.

Like their artistic colleagues a number of prominent scientists and inventors claim to have been guided or directed to significant theoretical or practical insights by voices. As an example, two men engaged in complex experiments involving photographic materials described how a voice experience at a crucial moment helped to point them in the right direction:

> The researches seemed to go in phases. An experimental result, or a momentary insight, would initiate fruitful progress. Then this would come to an end and the work would proceed desultorily, making little progress despite significant effort. On one such occasion, when one phase had been completed and Ted and Dennis seemed unable to find a way forward again, Ted woke up in the middle of the night having heard a voice clearly say, 'The secret is

in the liquids.' It then needed only a few minutes thought to realise that the way forward was, in fact, to work with the liquids.[62]

This kind of guidance, coming during a prolonged impasse in critical experimental or theoretical work, has occasionally played a key role in helping researchers to achieve an important scientific breakthrough.

11 *The Call of Vocation*

In everyday usage the word 'vocation' is usually understood to refer to a sense of having a strong interest in and aptitude for a particular career or occupation. However, as Carl Jung has pointed out, the way in which some people experience their vocational 'calling' is much closer to what was implied in the original meaning of the term:

> Vocation acts like a law of God from which there is no escape ... He *must* obey his own law, as if it were a daemon* whispering to him of new and wonderful paths. Anyone with a vocation hears the voice of the inner man: he is *called*. That is why the legends say that he possesses a private daemon who counsels him and whose mandates he must obey ... The original meaning of 'to have a vocation' is 'to be addressed by a voice'. The clearest examples of this are to be found in the avowals of the Old Testament prophets. That it is not just a quaint old-fashioned way of speaking is proved by the confessions of historical personalities such as Goethe and Napoleon, to mention only two familiar examples, who made no secret of their feeling of vocation. Vocation, or the feeling of it,

---

* In ancient Greece 'daimon' (also spelt 'daemon') referred to an attendant or in-dwelling inspirational spirit. Translated into Latin as *genii* it gave rise to the English word 'genius' which originally meant the tutelary deity or spirit presiding over a person's destiny. The modern term 'demon', which is usually used in a negative sense to refer solely to an *evil* spirit or devil, originated from a wrong translation and consequent misunderstanding of the original meaning of 'daimon'.

is not, however, the prerogative of great personalities; it is also appropriate to the small ones . . . [63]

While many people probably *feel* their vocational calling rather than hear it there are nevertheless those for whom the 'call' of an inner voice is a constant and powerful guiding influence. The Indian spiritual and political leader Mahatma Ghandi, for example, relied on such a voice for guidance throughout his life.[64] For some people a vocational call comes as a profoundly spiritual experience. As will be described in the next chapter, a number of important saints and other eminent religious figures have described the life-changing impact of receiving what they believed was a divine call to serve God's will. There are, on the other hand, many instances of people who have experienced an entirely secular vocational call via an inner voice. For example, the seminal French feminist writer Simone de Beauvoir has told of having such an experience shortly after returning home from an inspiring lecture which brought home to her for the first time the importance of serving the great community of humanity:

> I went back home in a state of exaltation; I was taking off my black coat and hat in the hall when I suddenly stood stock still; with my eyes fixed on the threadbare carpet, I heard an imperious voice within me saying: 'My life must be of service to humanity! Everything in my life must be of service!' I was stunned by the clear necessity of the call: innumerable tasks awaited me; it would need the whole strength of my being; if I allowed myself the slightest slackening of purpose, I would be betraying my trust and wronging humanity. 'Everything I do must be of service!' I told myself, with a tightening of the throat; it was a solemn vow, and I uttered it with as much feeling as if I had been pledging my whole future irrevocably in the face of heaven and earth . . . henceforward I made scrupulous use of every minute.[65]

Some people describe having heard a guiding inner voice at a time when they were suffering deep despair and uncertainty about their direction in life. M. Scott Peck, author of the international best-selling book, *The Road Less Travelled*, had such an experience as a young man feeling deeply confused and uncertain about whether or not to continue at the expensive boarding school his parents had chosen for him:

> If I returned to Exeter [school] I would be returning to all that was safe, secure, right, proper, constructive, proven and known. Yet it was not me. In the depths of my being I knew it was not my path. But what was my path? If I did not return, all that lay ahead was unknown, undetermined, unsafe, insecure, unsanctified, unpredictable. Anyone who would take such a path must be mad. I was terrified. But then, at the moment of my greatest despair, from my unconscious there came a sequence of words, like a strange disembodied oracle from a voice that was not mine: 'The only real security in life lies in relishing life's insecurity.' Even if it meant being crazy and out of step with all that seemed holy, I had decided to be me . . . I had taken the leap into the unknown. I had taken my destiny into my own hands.[66]

Although it is impossible to say just how many people may have had such experiences it is likely that they may be far more common than is usually realised. David Lukoff, a psychologist whose own experience of an audible call to become a healer led to a complete transformation of his professional life, believes that many mental health professionals may have been 'called' to their demanding and specialised field of work as a result of their own experience of profoundly unsettling emotional crises.[67] (Lukoff's experiences are described in Chapter Six.)

12 *Medical Disorders and Conditions*

The disturbances of physiological functioning associated with a wide range of medical disorders and conditions may facilitate the emergence of a variety of hallucinatory experiences. However, any hallucinations which occur in these circumstances are far more likely to involve visual (sight), tactile (touch), olfactory (smell) or gustatory (taste) experiences than auditory (hearing) ones.[68] Furthermore, if auditory hallucinations do occur in association with physical disorders they usually have an elementary or primitive quality, i.e. the affected person hears noises such as buzzing, humming, ringing, and so on. Such experiences also tend to be rather fleeting, fragmentary and changeable in nature, and they generally accompany hallucinations in one or more of the other sensory modalities.

It is well-known that fevers, with their associated elevation of brain temperature, are often accompanied by hallucination-like experiences. In fact, it is no exaggeration to say that every human being is only ever a few degrees away from experiences of this kind! It has been observed that hyperventilation (i.e. prolonged rapid and deep breathing) may facilitate the occurrence of auditory and visual hallucinations in some people.[69] On the other hand, a lowered respiratory rate, or even a complete holding of the breath, has been reported to lead to the onset of auditory hallucinations in certain persons.[70] Medical conditions which effect the central nervous system can produce a range of hallucinatory phenomena. Thus, hallucinations have been reported to occur in association with neurological disorders such as the post-concussion syndrome, migraine, various types of intracranial tumours (especially those located in the temporal lobe), viral encephalitis, and temporal lobe epilepsy.[71]

Hallucinations of various kinds can also occur as side-effects or toxic effects of a wide range of commonly prescribed medical drugs including sedatives and hypnotics, psychostimulants (e.g. amphetamines), psychotropics (e.g. anti-depressants, lithium carbonate), cardiovascular drugs (e.g. anti-hypertensives), local anaesthetics, hormones (e.g. corticosteroids), analgesics (e.g. aspirin), anti-inflammatory drugs, anti-infection agents (e.g. antibiotics), and anti-neoplastic drugs. Even the neuroleptic drugs (also known as 'major tranquillisers') which are often used for the purposes of controlling or eliminating psychotic symptoms have been known to intensify hallucinations or elicit new ones in people who are hypersensitive to their anticholinergic properties.[72] An hallucinatory syndrome is one of the most common and well-known complications of long-term drug therapy of Parkinson's disease. The hallucinations typically consist of formed images of people or animals, and often involve persons familiar to the patient such as absent or dead friends or relatives whose distinct and familiar voices are sometimes distinctly heard.[73]

Some Famous Voice Hearers

History reveals that a considerable number of exemplary individuals have heard voices. Amongst them may be included the likes of Sigmund Freud, Carl Jung, Mahatma Gandhi, Socrates, William Blake, Martin Luther King Jr, Elisabeth Kübler-Ross, and the classical music composer Robert Schumann.[74] Within the religious and spiritual context numerous examples could be also be cited including Moses, Jesus Christ, Saint Paul, Saint Teresa, Saint Augustine, Saint Francis, Joan of Arc, Luther, John Bunyan, George Fox (founder of the Quakers), Joseph Smith (founder of the Mormons), Mohammed (founder of Islam), and the Swedish philosopher Emanuel Swedenborg. The specific experiences of some of these influential persons are discussed in more detail in later sections of this book. However, in order to illustrate the wide range of different voice experiences that can occur, those of Freud, Socrates and Jung will be briefly described here.

Sigmund Freud, the Viennese psychiatrist who founded psychoanalysis early this century, has described having often heard his name being called aloud when he was wide awake. So vivid was the experience that on several occasions he was moved to investigate whether there was any veridical aspect to the experience, although he says he never found any:

> During the days when I was living alone in a foreign city . . . I quite often heard my name suddenly called by an unmistakable and beloved voice; I then noted down the exact moment of the hallucination and made anxious enquiries of those at home about what had happened at that time. Nothing had happened.[75]

The renowned philosopher of ancient Greece, Socrates, claimed that for most of his life he heard an admonitory inner voice to which he attributed a divine origin. The voice never told him what to do but simply advised him not to follow certain courses of action which were not in his best interest. Socrates insisted that the voice, which he believed to be that of a God (or 'daemon'), was never wrong in the advice and guidance it provided him:

> You may have heard me say that a sort of divine thing, a spirit agency . . . comes into my experience . . . Ever since my boyhood I have had experience of a certain voice,

which, when it comes to me, always forbids me to do something which I am going to do, but never commands me to do anything; it is this which opposes my following a political career.[76]

Such was the confidence that Socrates had in this inner voice that he followed its dictates and did not prepare a defence for himself when he was eventually placed on trial. When he was found guilty and asked to choose between exile and death he chose to die, explaining that he did so because 'the oracle made no sign of opposition'.

The Swiss psychiatrist Carl Gustav Jung had numerous voice experiences throughout his long and distinguished professional career. Jung, who was originally a close colleague of Freud, eventually founded his own unique approach to depth psychology which he termed 'Analytical Psychology'. For Jung, the inner worlds of the imagination and dreams were richly informative regarding the secret contents and dynamics of the human psyche. Many of Jung's most important psychological insights came to him as a result of interactions with figures that presented themselves to him spontaneously in his dreams and fantasies. During the especially turbulent phase of his life he referred to as his 'confrontation with the unconscious' Jung had a number of deeply moving encounters with imaginal beings which arose from his unconscious, the most important of whom he named 'Philemon'. In an experience recounted in his autobiographical memoir, *Memories, Dreams, Reflections*, Jung has described how he engaged in animated conversation with Philemon and the many other autonomous fantasy figures that were to become his companions and teachers:

> In my fantasies I held conversations with him, and he said things which I had not consciously thought. For I observed clearly that it was he who spoke, not I ... He was a mysterious figure to me. At times he seemed to me quite real, as if he were a living personality. I went walking up and down the garden with him, and to me he was what the Indians call a guru.[77]

Over a period of many years Jung cultivated and sustained valuable creative relationships with Philemon and other imaginal beings. He eventually developed the therapeutic technique he called 'active imagination' as a result of his efforts to fully engage and relate with the personified figures of his fantasies and dreams. (Chapter Nine contains a detailed discussion of the use of active imagination to work with voice experiences.)

Conclusion

The information presented in this chapter serves as a broad introduction to the fascinating subject of hearing voices. It shows quite clearly that voice experiences can take a wide variety of forms and occur in a vast range of different circumstances. Many readers will undoubtedly have recognised in these pages accounts of experiences they themselves have had or that someone known to them has described.

It is unfortunate that, in Western societies at least, a lack of understanding of these kinds of experiences has led to a widespread fear of them which has many undesirable consequences. As an example, despite the fact that they are described as being *helpful* by most people who have them, the voices and visions which often accompany bereavement are generally hidden from others and may therefore contribute to needless worry and apprehension. By way of contrast, the more enlightened attitudes that exist toward such experiences in many non-Western societies result in an acceptance of them as a natural part of the grieving process which can be openly shared. Nor are bereaved persons alone in terms of being privy to experiences about which we still have precious little understanding. Sadly, it is not unusual for the extraordinary reports of those who have come close to death to be treated with suspicion despite the fact that huge numbers of similar experiences have been reported by persons whose honesty and integrity cannot reasonably be in doubt. These phenomena warrant serious consideration. While the near-death experience does not in itself prove the existence of a spiritual after-life it raises many important questions. If a NDE is not a glimpse of a state of consciousness that continues after ordinary physical life has ended, what is it? It is rather ironic that, while sensory phenomena such as voices and visions represent key aspects of the NDE, the total experience itself appears to open a door onto vistas which extend well beyond the sensory and material.

This chapter has made it clear that inner voice experiences are not confined to mentally disturbed persons. This in itself will be challenging to some. Perhaps even more challenging is the fact that a number of reputable studies have shown that voice hearing experiences of a kind often considered to be characteristic of schizophrenia (e.g. voices repeating the hearer's thoughts aloud) are *frequently* reported by persons who are, for all intents and purposes, mentally normal. The implications of this will be taken up in later chapters in which the voices of schizophrenia and other mental disorders are discussed in detail.

Mental disorders of various kinds undoubtedly constitute one of the major realms of human experience in which voice hearing often occurs, though even here many misunderstandings have developed concerning their complex nature and origin. For the moment attention will be devoted to another of the vast and important areas of human experience with which voices are frequently associated: the domain of spirituality.

Chapter Two

VOICES AND SPIRITUALITY

*Let us silence the desires and importunings of the flesh and
the vainglorious fantasies of our imagination, so that we can
freely hear what the spirit is saying. Let our ears be attuned
to the voice that is heard above the vault of heaven, for the
Spirit of Life is always speaking to our souls.*

– Julian of Vezelay[78]

The experience of hearing a voice or voices to which a supernatural
origin is attributed has been enormously important throughout
human history. Whether occurring on their own or in association
with visions or other sensory experiences such voices inevitably
have a powerful effect upon the hearer. Whilst there are undoubtedly many among the vast range of purportedly spiritual voice
experiences which are actually fanciful products of the hearer's
imagination or some other form of sensory deception, there are
nevertheless some which are profoundly important to those who
hear them:

> These bring wisdom to the simple and ignorant, sudden
> calm to those who were tormented by doubts. They flood
> the personality with new light: accompany conversion, or
> the passage from one spiritual state to another: arrive at
> moments of indecision, bringing with them authoritative
> commands or counsels, opposed to the inclination of the
> self: confer a convinced knowledge of some department of
> the spiritual life before unknown.[79]

In a significant number of instances spiritual voice experiences have
led directly to the founding of influential religious movements with
huge numbers of adherents. Indeed, it is no exaggeration to say that
the origins of some of the world's greatest religious traditions are
to be found in deeply moving inner experiences involving voices:

The history of the world's major religions makes it clear that saints, sages, prophets, and teachers (such as Moses, Mohammed, and Teresa of Avila) have relied heavily on the inner voice as their inspiration, their guidance, and their authority. The inner voice experiences of these men and women have had a tremendous impact on our world.[80]

The following overview of a wide range of religious traditions and spiritual experiences which have involved hearing voices reveals just how important this phenomenon has been in all human cultures throughout the ages.

Ancient Civilisations

Throughout ancient Egypt, Rome, Babylon, Tibet and Greece the advice and guidance of oracular voices was sought and highly valued. For more than a thousand years in Greece oracles were called upon when important decisions needed to be made. A variety of means were relied upon to obtain advice and guidance from these oracles. In the early days it was widely believed that at certain sacred sites it was possible for the supplicant to directly hear the voice of a god. In later times it was more common for the divine message to be mediated through the agency of a specially appointed priest or priestess who heard the voice of the god and relayed its message to others. Whilst oracles were often consulted for advice regarding worldly affairs they also provided highly sought after guidance in religious and spiritual matters. Indeed, such was the esteem in which they were held that Plato referred to the oracle of Apollo at Delphi as 'the interpreter of religion to all mankind'.[81] There were many oracles in addition to the famous one at Delphi. Thus, the voice of Zeus was heard at Dodona, whilst Pan had an oracle at Acacesium, and the goddess Artemis was heard to speak through priests at Ephesus. The most long-lasting of the direct oracles, whose voice was heard without any intermediary priest or priestess, was that of Trophonius at Lebadea. In order to consult Trophonius it was necessary for the supplicant to descend and remain alone in a dark cavern consecrated to this god.

The Judaeo-Christian Tradition

The Judaeo-Christian tradition, as exemplified in the Old and the New Testaments of the Bible, is replete with descriptions of divine or demonic beings speaking directly to humans. In the Book of Genesis, for example, it is stated that on the sixth day of creation God spoke to Adam and Eve, the new beings He had created in His image (Genesis, 1:27–28, RSV); shortly thereafter He gave Adam commandments regarding his responsibilities in the garden of Eden (Genesis, 2:16–17).

The Old Testament

The God of the Old Testament promised that He would reveal Himself to human beings through visions and voices, and to numerous of the Old Testament heroes and prophets He did so, though to the Hebrew prophet Moses it is said He granted a special dispensation. The book of Exodus records the well-known instance in which God spoke to Moses from out of a burning bush, whilst elsewhere it is said that 'the Lord used to speak to Moses face to face, as a man speaks to his friend' (Exodus, 33:11, RSV). Historically the most significant incident in which God spoke to Moses is probably the one that occurred on Mount Sinai when God dictated to him the Ten Commandments (Exodus, 34:27–28, RSV). This event had profound ramifications for the Jewish people and eventually for the entire Christian world as well.

The New Testament

The New Testament contains many accounts of incidents in which an individual hears supernatural voices. It is said, for example, that angels spoke directly to Mary (Luke 1:28–30, RSV), Joseph (Matthew 1:20), Zechariah (Luke 1:13) and Mary Magdalene (John 20:13). On at least three important occasions Jesus Himself heard a supernatural voice speaking to Him. The first of these incidents occurred following His baptism in the River Jordan (Mark, 1:10–11). Soon afterwards Jesus was led by the Spirit into the wilderness where He was tempted by the devil who spoke to Him (Matthew, 4:3–10). According to Matthew's gospel, Moses and Elijah appeared during Jesus' transfiguration and spoke with Him (Matthew, 17:3).

Then, it is said, a bright cloud overshadowed them and a voice from the cloud said, 'This is my beloved Son, with whom I am well pleased; listen to Him.' (Matthew, 17:5).*

One of the most famous incidents in the New Testament, and one which was to prove a decisive turning-point in the history of the early Christian church, involved the experience of Saul (later to become St Paul) who heard the voice of Jesus on the road to Damascus:

> Now as he journeyed he approached Damascus, and suddenly a light from heaven flashed about him. And he fell to the ground and heard a voice saying to him, 'Saul, Saul, why do you persecute me?' And he said, 'Who are you, Lord?' And he said, 'I am Jesus, whom you are persecuting; but rise and enter the city, and you will be told what you are to do.' The men who were travelling with him stood speechless, hearing the voice but seeing no one.
> (Acts, 9:3–7, RSV)

It is said that following this experience Paul's conversion to Christianity was complete, and he thereafter became the greatest champion of its evangelical mission.†

The last book of the New Testament contains a detailed account of the revelation received by the apostle John on the island of Patmos. Commonly known as 'The Apocalypse', this graphic description of the final days of the world was revealed to John in a series of mysterious visions. According to John's own account, in this revelation the voice of Jesus 'was like the sound of many waters' (Revelation,1:15).

---

* Interestingly, Peter, James and John, the three disciples who were with Jesus at the time, also heard God's voice speaking from the cloud. This was a *collective* voice experience and it is written that they fell on their faces and were filled with awe in response to it. The voice experience of Saul (St Paul) on the road to Damascus was also apparently a collective one.

† The sanity of those who have profound spiritual experiences is often questioned by others who are rather more sceptically-minded. Paul was no exception. When he described his experience to the Roman governor Festus he was told: 'Paul, you are mad; your great learning is turning you mad.' (Acts, 26:24, RSV)

Early Christian Saints and Mystics

A study of the lives of the great Christian saints and mystics reveals that a wide range of experiences involving voices (with or without any accompanying visions) were common among these exalted individuals. Indeed, in his classic study of the psychology of religious experience William James recognised that the mystic temperament lends itself to these kinds of experiences:

> The whole array of Christian saints and heresiarchs, including the greatest, the Barnards, the Loyolas, the Luthers, the Foxes, the Wesleys, had their visions, voices, rapt conditions, guiding impressions, and 'openings'. They had these things because they had exalted sensibility, and to such things persons of exalted sensibility are liable. In such liability there lie . . . consequences for theology.[82]

It is noteworthy that in Western Europe during the Middle Ages a spiritual world-view was so prevalent that there was simply no concept of auditory or visual 'hallucinations' in the modern sense. Rather, people were thought to be capable of receiving revelations or seeing visions of a supernatural kind. Thus, any person who heard voices was simply considered to have had a true experience involving contact with divine or demonic beings or agencies.[83] It is noteworthy, however, that all the great mystics warned their disciples to be wary about placing too much importance on these kinds of experiences and urged them to be extremely cautious in accepting them at face value as 'messages from God'. Nevertheless, as the eminent scholar of mysticism Evelyn Underhill has noted:

> These visions and voices are such frequent accompaniments of the mystic life, that they cannot be ignored. The messengers of the invisible world knock persistently at the doors of the senses: and not only at those which refer to hearing and to sight. In other words, supersensual intuitions – the contact between man's finite being and the Infinite Being in which it is immersed – can express themselves by means of almost any kind of sensory automatism ... All those so-called 'hallucinations of the senses' which appear in the history of mysticism must, then, be considered soberly, frankly, and without prejudice

in the course of our inquiry into the psychology of man's quest of the Real.[84]

A number of important Christian saints have themselves written extensively on the subject of voices, and especially on their proper place in religious and spiritual life. Notable among them are St John of the Cross (1542–1591), whose *Ascent of Mount Carmel* is considered a spiritual classic, and his teacher St Teresa of Avila (1515–1582), considered by many to be one of the most profound teachers in the history of Christianity and the first woman to be proclaimed a Doctor of the Catholic Church (by Pope Paul VI in 1970). Teresa dealt at length with various aspects of the phenomenon of voices (which she calls 'locutions') in what is regarded as her greatest work, *The Interior Castle*. She was especially concerned to distinguish between those locutions which are considered to be genuine since they come from God or His saints, and those which are considered false because they come from the imagination or the devil. So important did Teresa consider this subject that she devoted an entire chapter of *The Interior Castle* to it:

There are many kinds of locutions [voices] given to the soul. Some seem to come from outside oneself; others, from deep within the interior part of the soul; others, from the superior part; and some are so exterior that they come through the sense of hearing, for it seems there is a spoken word. Sometimes, and often, the locution can be an illusion, especially in persons with a weak imagination or in those who are melancholic, I mean who suffer noticeably from melancholy. In my opinion no attention should be paid to these latter two kinds of persons even if they say they see and hear and understand. But neither should one disturb these persons by telling them their locutions come from the devil; one must listen to them as sick persons. The prioress or confessor to whom they relate their locutions should tell them to pay no attention to such experiences ... all the kinds [of locutions] I mentioned can be from God or from the devil or from one's own imagination. If I can manage to do so, I shall give ... the signs as to when they come from these different sources and when they are dangerous;

for there are many souls among prayerful people who hear them.[85]

The traditional classification of mystical voice experiences (which are also referred to as 'locutions' or 'auditions') recognises three main types:[86]

(1) 'Intellectual' Locutions: these involve the experience of an 'immediate' or inarticulate voice whose words or statements are perceived directly by the person's intellect without the aid of the external sense of hearing or the imagination. St Teresa described these locutions as being heard 'with the ears of the soul'. Thus, religious mystics and persons who believe themselves to be in direct communication with spiritual guidance sometimes describe:

> a voice which is yet soundless, which utters the 'language of the soul' inside them, and which they hear by means of a 'sixth sense', and without any apparent participation of the ear.[87]

(2) 'Imaginative' Locutions: these involve the experience of hearing a distinct interior voice which is perfectly articulate but recognised as speaking only within the person's own mind. They may occur during sleep or whilst awake.

(3) 'Corporeal' (Auricular) Locutions: these involve hearing an exterior voice which belongs to a being that may either be seen or invisible. The voice is experienced as speaking externally to the person and is heard by their outer ear. The voices that were heard by the well known saint, Joan of Arc (see below) were of this kind. Because they involve 'exterior words', these experiences have been regarded by some mystics with a degree of suspicion and dislike. Regarding such locutions St John of the Cross said, 'The more corporal they are, the less certain is their divine origin.'[88] The Roman Catholic Church nevertheless holds that even these experiences may sometimes have a supernatural origin:

> Auricular locutions are words perceived by the bodily sense of hearing, and are generally caused by supernaturally produced acoustical vibrations. They sometimes seem to emanate from a vision or a religious object such as a statue or crucifix. As extraordinary phenomena they could be caused by God or the devil or proceed from natural causes.[89]

If voice experiences which originate in the imagination are excluded there nevertheless remain some which exert a very profound and positive influence on the spiritual life of the hearer. There are several ways in which such genuine spiritual experiences may be mediated by voices:

(a) Conversion and Vocation

The term 'vocation' originally referred to the experience of being called by an inner voice. The lives of a number of notable religious persons bear witness to the fact that some of them did indeed *literally* hear such a call and respond to it in a life-changing way. The most famous example of this phenomenon is undoubtedly that of Saul (later St Paul) on the road to Damascus (described earlier). St Teresa herself has described how her faith was awakened by an inner voice which she heard as she was reading the *Confessions* of St Augustine. St Francis of Assisi (1182–1226), who is known as the father of Italian mysticism, was converted by a voice experience of the corporeal type. Following a prolonged period of struggle in which he felt torn between the life of the world and the call of the spirit Francis one day found himself in an emotionally divided state praying in a crumbling and derelict church:

> And whilst he was thus moved ... the painted image of Christ Crucified spoke to him from out its painted lips. And, calling him by his name, 'Francis,' it said, 'go, repair My house, the which as thou seest is falling into decay.' And Francis trembled, being utterly amazed, and almost as it were carried away by these words. And he prepared to obey for he was wholly set on the fulfilling of this commandment ... In a moment of time, Francis's whole universe has suffered complete rearrangement ... Not for a moment does he think of disobeying the imperative voice which speaks to him from a higher plane of reality and demands the sacrifice of his career.[90]

(b) Guidance, Direction and Inspiration

Inner voices inspired and guided the spiritual lives of a number of the saints. Indeed, the entire religious career of some was given over to obediently following the instruction of their voices. St Teresa, for example, was subject to direction by her locutions in every aspect of her life:

> St Teresa's mystic life was governed by voices: her active career as a foundress was much guided by them. They advised her in small things as in great. Often they interfered with her plans, ran counter to her personal judgement, forbade a foundation on which she was set, or commanded one which appeared imprudent or impossible. They concerned themselves with journeys, with the purchase of houses; they warned her of coming events. As her mystical life matured, Teresa seems to have learned to discriminate those locutions on which action should properly be based. She seldom resisted them, though it constantly happened that the action on which they insisted seemed the height of folly: and though they frequently involved her in hardships and difficulties, she never had cause to regret this reliance upon decrees which she regarded as coming direct from God, and which certainly did emanate from a life greater than her own.[91]

Undoubtedly the most famous of the saints who were subject to the guidance of voices was Joan of Arc (1412–1431).[92] Voices appear to have influenced her life in two distinct phases. The first began at the age of thirteen with a sudden revelation of a corporeal voice which she believed to be that of the archangel Michael who told her that henceforth two other saints, Catherine and Margaret, would give her instructions that she must follow. Joan initially heard the voices two or three times a week and at this stage they simply instructed and guided her spiritually and consolidated her faith by exhorting her to live a good life and to pray fervently. Later, the voices ceased giving her general instructions regarding a virtuous life and began issuing orders which were to lead to the actions for which she became famous. At the specific behest of her voices Joan eventually led the French army to victory over the English, an event which altered the course of European history and ultimately the future of the entire Western world. For at least six or seven years of her short life Joan received continuous instruction, guidance, and consolation from the voices which, even at the moment of her martyrdom, she insisted came to her from God. There is little doubt that without them her life and the lives of many others would have been very different. St Joan of Arc exemplifies the fact that in some cases the experience of voices has consequences which extend well beyond their immediate impact on the hearer's own inner life.

(c) Instruction and Illumination

For many of the saints and mystics it was by means of direct instruction provided by voices that their most profound spiritual insights were developed. For example, Abbess Hildegard of Bingen (1098–1179), arguably one of the most remarkable creative individuals of the Middle Ages, said that all of her voluminous writings were dictated to her by the Holy Ghost:

> I hear these things not with the bodily ears, nor the thoughts of my mind, nor perceive them through any combination of the five senses, but entirely within my soul.[93]

Some individuals have been privy to revelations which came to them in the form of an inner dialogue. In such 'intimate colloquies between Divine Reality and the Soul' various spiritually edifying instruction have sometimes been received:

> The self, wholly absorbed by the intimate sense of divine companionship, receives its messages in the form of 'distinct interior words'; as of an alien voice, speaking within the mind with such an accent of validity and spontaneity as to leave no room for doubt as to its character . . . [The hearer] recognising the Voice as personal and distinct from its own soul naturally enters into a communion which has an almost conversational character, replies to questions or asks others in its turn: and in this dramatic style the content of its intuitions is gradually expressed.[94]

An important example of this form of illumination is provided in *The Imitation of Christ*, a spiritual classic attributed to Thomas à Kempis (1380–1471). In the third book of this work the author discusses the experience of 'The Voice of Christ in the Heart, Speaking to the Faithful Soul'. The Lord himself has promised, says

Thomas, that 'The man to whom I speak will soon be wise and make great spiritual progress.'[95]

(d) Assurance

Whilst the virtues of faith have always been strongly emphasised within the Christian tradition, tangible experiences which help to strengthen and consolidate spiritual beliefs have always been keenly sought after. As William James has noted, the experience of voices (or visions) may have the effect of strengthening the hearer's faith in those aspects of the spiritual world which remain hidden to the physical senses:

> Beliefs are strengthened wherever automatisms corroborate them. Incursions from beyond the transmarginal region have a peculiar power to increase conviction. The inchoate sense of presence is infinitely stronger than conception, but strong as it may be, it seldom equals the evidence of hallucination. Saints who actually see or hear their Saviour reach the acme of assurance.[96]

Joan of Arc's story exemplifies this. Following her betrayal by the French and capture by the English she was imprisoned, interrogated and eventually condemned to death as a witch by the Inquisition. Nevertheless, she clung to the comforting presence of her spiritual guides. Such was the strength of her conviction that even the most extreme measures taken by the Inquisitors in an effort to force her to repudiate her voices all failed. As she stood upon the funeral pyre in her very last moments her faith remained unwavering. At the moment of her death Joan still insisted that everything she had done had been at God's command and that her voices were undoubtedly His direct revelations to her.

Even for St Teresa, concerned as she was with the discernment of true and false voices, there were certain prized experiences which, by their very nature, convinced the hearer that they could *only* have their source in God:

> There is another way in which the Lord speaks to the soul – for I hold that it is very definitely from Him ... The locution takes place in such intimate depths and a person with the ears of the soul seems to hear those words from

the Lord Himself so clearly and so in secret that this very way in which they are heard together with the acts that the vision itself produces, assures the person and gives him certitude that the devil can have no part to play in the locution. Wonderful effects are left so that the soul may believe; at least there is assurance that the locution doesn't come from the imagination.[97]

(e) Prophecy

A number of saints claim to have been told by their voices of things that would occur in the future. The most famous example of this phenomenon is undoubtedly the Revelation of St John which comprises the last book of the Bible. St Teresa also said that she was forewarned of coming events by her voices. For several years following the moment she was first instructed by her voices to begin the campaign to free France from the English, Joan of Arc received numerous revelations regarding future events involving herself and others. In many instances it seems to have been these prophecies which enabled her to plan and direct her successful political and military strategies. Joan never felt in any doubt regarding the ultimate outcome of her struggle since her voices had told her that the liberation of France was assured. It is recorded that the voices even predicted her eventual capture by the English army.

Modern Christian Religious Leaders

Many examples could be given of individuals in more recent times to whom voices have provided guidance and instruction. In some cases these experiences have led to the founding of influential new religious movements. A good example can be found in George Fox (1624–1691), founder of the Religious Society of Friends (who are also known as 'Quakers'). In his youth Fox experienced a prolonged period of torment and unrest during which he searched the Scriptures and wandered about the country vainly seeking answers to his burning spiritual questions. In his *Journal* he tells how the end of this search came about quite suddenly:

> I fasted much, walked abroad in solitary places many days, and often took my Bible, and sat in hollow trees and

lonesome places until night came on; and frequently in the night walked mournfully about by myself; for I was a man of sorrows in the time of the first workings of the Lord in me ... As I had forsaken the priests, so I left the separate preachers also, and those called the most experienced people; for I saw there was none among them all that could speak to my condition. And when all my hopes in them and in all men were gone, so that I had nothing outwardly to help me, nor could tell what to do, then, oh then, I heard a voice which said, 'There is one, even Jesus Christ, that can speak to thy condition', and when I heard it my heart did leap for joy. Then the Lord let me see why there was none upon the earth that could speak to my condition.[98]

Following his conversion Fox wandered throughout England preaching and following the commands of God which he heard as a voice. To this day, traditional Quaker services are held in silence so that members of the congregation can listen for 'the still, small voice within'.

The vision which Joseph Smith claims to have beheld when he was barely fifteen years old ultimately led to the founding of the Church of Jesus Christ of Latter-day Saints ('Mormons'). Like George Fox before him, Smith had also been seeking guidance regarding which religious sect he should join. This is his own account of the awesome revelation he experienced:

Thick darkness gathered around me ... just at this moment of great alarm, I saw a pillar of light exactly over my head, above the brightness of the sun, which descended gradually until it fell upon me. [Then] I saw two personages, whose brightness and glory defy all description, standing above me in the air. One of them spake unto me, calling me by name, and said, pointing to the other – 'This is my beloved Son, hear him!' ... I asked the personages who stood above me in the light which of the sects was right ... I was answered that I must join none of them, for they were all wrong ... many other things did he say unto me, which I cannot write at this time.[99]

Joseph Smith claimed that he received many other revelations following this initial one and that he was directly guided and instructed in a new Christian teaching. This instruction culminated in the formal establishment of the new faith in 1830. It remains the official doctrine of the Mormon Church that God spoke in person to Joseph Smith and that similar divine revelations of God's will continue to this day.

Contemporary Religious Experience

Voice experiences of a spiritually profound and edifying kind are not the sole prerogative of medieval saints and mystics, nor of those exalted souls who were responsible for founding new religious movements. It appears that many ordinary men and women have had such experiences, though they usually remain a completely private and personal matter. In his famous study of the psychology of religious conversion Professor Edwin Starbuck noted that it was not at all rare for a person to hear a voice in the moments preceding their conversion.[100] For example, at this particular time one man heard a voice coming from outside himself which said, 'Believe in me, for I am God.' It appears that the 'call of a divine voice' has led many people to their Christian vocation. The following account illustrates the way in which one person's decision to join the ministry followed his experience of such a call:

> The great experience that led me to be ordained was when I was about seventeen. I went on a lonely walking tour [and] one morning I was drawing near the ruins of Rievaulx Abbey . . . I sensed a wonderful atmosphere of quiet peace, and then heard a most entrancing voice which in one way seemed external and yet in another from deep down within me, calling me to be ordained. I saw nothing, yet I was convinced it was Christ Himself and he desired me like Andrew and Peter to rise up and follow Him and be ordained. With the voice came the Inner Conviction that Christ would make all things possible.[101]

Some people who already have a Christian faith claim that their own specific 'calling' was revealed to them by a voice. Briege McKenna, an Irish nun renowned for her remarkable spiritual healing powers, claims to have been called to her healing ministry by Jesus himself:

I had been in the chapel about five minutes when suddenly this extraordinary stillness descended on the chapel – it was like a cloud, like a fog. A voice said, 'Briege.' I turned to look toward the door because the voice was so clear it sounded as though someone had come into the chapel. No one was there, but I was very conscious that someone was present. The voice said to me as I turned back to the tabernacle, 'You have my gift of healing. Go and use it.' I remember looking at my hands. It felt as though I had touched an electrical outlet.[102]

Some contemporary spiritual voice experiences have awakened the curiosity and interest of large numbers of people. For example, since 1981 when six teenage children claim that they began receiving revelatory messages directly from the Virgin Mary, Medjugorje has become a revered holy site for worshippers from all over the world. The lives of countless numbers of people have been deeply affected as a result of these apparitions, about which Pope John Paul II has spoken favourably on many occasions.[103]

The Islamic Tradition

According to Islamic tradition the prophet Mohammed, as the last founder of a world religion, received his divine mandate directly from God through the agency of the archangel Gabriel (known in Arabic as 'Jibril'). Born in Mecca in 570 AD, Mohammed was in his fortieth year when this revelation took place. During the holy month of Ramadan he had gone to a cave on Mount Hira near Mecca to seek communion with God in fasting, prayer and solitary meditation. It was there that the supernatural messenger first came to him:

As Mohammed, in the silent watches of the night, lay wrapped in his mantle, he heard a voice calling upon him. Uncovering his head, a flood of light broke upon him of such intolerable splendour that he swooned away. On regaining his senses he beheld an angel in a human form, which, approaching from a distance, displayed a silken cloth covered with written characters. 'Read!' said the angel. 'I know not how to read!' replied Mohammed. 'Read!' repeated the angel, 'in the name of the Lord, who has created all things; who created man from a clot of blood. Read in the name of the Most High, who taught man the use of the pen; who sheds on his soul the ray of knowledge and teaches him what before he knew not.' Upon this Mohammed felt his understanding illumined with celestial light and read what was written on the cloth, which contained the decrees of God, as afterwards promulgated in the Koran. When he had finished the perusal the heavenly messenger announced: 'Oh, Mohammed, of a verity thou art the prophet of God! And I am his Angel Gabriel!'[104]

It is said that Mohammed, being unfamiliar with such experiences, did not immediately understand the nature of this call. He returned home, wondering if he was suffering from some kind of fever or, worse still, if he had not been visited by an evil spirit. Soon afterwards, however, he had another meeting with the angelic messenger. During this second encounter many of his problems were solved and his questions answered and his earlier fears and doubts were soon allayed. After a longer interval Mohammed was once again visited by Gabriel who revealed that he (Mohammed) had been chosen by God to be His Last Messenger on earth. The Koran, which is the Holy Book of Islam, is believed by Muslims to be a faithful record of the Divine message as revealed to the Prophet Mohammed through the direct revelation of the angel Gabriel. In modern times the pursuit of direct contact with the spiritual realm is a widely accepted practice within the mystical Sufi tradition of Islam.

Non-Denominational Spiritual Experiences

People sometimes hear voices as part of a spiritual experience which occurs outside the context of any particular formal religious belief system. Several studies have suggested that this phenomenon is not at all rare. For example, in a comprehensive survey conducted by the Religious Experiences Research Unit at Oxford University in which numerous first-hand accounts of religious experiences were collected, 431 out of 3,000 respondents (7%) reported having heard voices.[105] The authors of the survey commented that these seemed to be entirely self-vindicating, primary experiences whose reality for the subject was beyond question. The experiences reported seemed to fall into two main types: 'voices calming' and 'voices guiding'. The following is an example of the calming type of voice experience:

> Gradually I became aware of this power and began really to court it. It has come to me often – once in a dream – as light, warmth, comfort and love past understanding. It has walked with me and sometimes I hear something or someone calling my name.[106]

Some of the survey respondents said that the voice they heard seemed to come from within themselves whilst others said that it originated in the outer world. Some felt that it was both at once. In many cases this voice experience had a great religious significance for the hearer and often made a very profound impression upon them.

The results of a number of other studies lend support to these findings and suggest that a variety of voice experiences having a religious or spiritual nature are widespread in the human population. In a recent study of 375 college students, for example, 43 (11%) said that they had heard God's voice.[107] This experience specifically involved hearing God speak 'as a real voice' not simply knowing it as something in one's heart. The psychologists who conducted this research concluded that these kinds of 'normal auditory hallucinations' probably play a significant role in the development and reinforcement of many people's religious and supernatural belief systems. In another recent study of 186 people who reported hearing voices it was found that nearly half believed their voices to be 'gods' or 'spirits' of some kind.[108] Some felt their voices were a friend or a guide and tutor, whilst others believed themselves to be paranormally gifted ('clairaudient'). The author of one study of 'inner voice experiences' identified a group of persons for whom inner voices served as 'channels toward a higher self'.[109] Many of these persons felt that their inner voice was related to intuition and they consistently saw it as part of the spiritual dimension of their being. Voice experiences of this kind appear to have provided an important source of spiritual guidance to many people, including some very famous ones:

> Mahatma Gandhi, both a spiritual and political leader, relied on 'inner voice' as his primary guidance in life.

Gandhi described the inner voice as full of power and authority. A year before his death the voice told him, 'You are on the right track, move neither to your left, nor right, but keep to the straight and narrow.'[110]

Many examples can be found of voices providing spiritual comfort or guidance to persons in situations of extreme physical and emotional distress. There are war-time reports, for example, of torpedoed sailors immersed in the sea for hours who conversed with an audible God.[111] Silviu Craciunas, who suffered imprisonment and torture as a member of the Romanian post-war resistance movement, has described how, when he had reached his lowest physical and spiritual ebb, a 'personality' appeared to him in his cell in the form of a wise old brahmin who claimed to be a manifestation of Craciunas' inner spirit. Over many weeks the conversations that Craciunas had with the brahmin nurtured his spirit and provided him with the strength he needed to survive his painful ordeal.[112] A somewhat similar experience occurred to the famous sixteenth century Florentine sculptor Benvenuto Cellini whilst he was imprisoned in Rome by order of the Pope. As he contemplated suicide Cellini suddenly felt that a divine power in the form of a 'guardian angel' had intervened to prevent him from harming himself:

> At first I dreamed that God had saved me but as my sufferings continued and I once more was faced with suicide, the invisible being that had prevented my laying violent hands upon myself came to me, still invisible, but spoke with an audible voice. It shook me, made me rouse up and said, 'Benvenuto, Benvenuto, lose no time. Raise your heart to God in fervent devotion and cry to him with the utmost vehemence.'[113]

Emanuel Swedenborg, the Swedish polymath and teacher of William Blake, claimed to have held long conversations with what he believed were angels. He eventually developed his elaborate cosmology of spirit-worlds as a result of conversing with these angels in the guise of inner voices:

> Angels talk with each other just as men do in the world, and on various subjects, as on domestic matters, and on matters of civil, moral, and spiritual life. And there is no

difference except that their talk is more intelligent than that of men, because it is from more interior thought. I have been permitted to associate with them frequently, and to talk with them as friend with friend, and sometimes as stranger with stranger; and as I was then in a state like theirs I knew no otherwise than that I was talking with men on the earth. Angelic speech, the same as human speech, has distinct words; it is also audibly uttered and heard; for angels, like men, have mouth, tongue, and ears, and an atmosphere in which the sound of their speech is articulated, although it is a spiritual atmosphere adapted to angels who are spiritual.[114]

Spiritualism

Spiritualism is a philosophy which incorporates the belief that there exist departed human spirits with which it is possible to communicate. So-called 'mediums' allegedly have the ability to contact such spirits at will during seances or at other times, and some claim to be able to speak with them and hear their spoken replies to questions put to them by other people. Carl Jung studied the activities of a young woman medium as part of his pioneering parapsychological research early this century. When he questioned her about her elaborate spiritualistic experiences he discovered that she was totally convinced of their reality:

I do not know if what the spirits say and teach me is true, nor do I know if they really are the people they call themselves; but that my spirits exist is beyond question. I see them before me, I can touch them. I speak to them about everything I wish as naturally as I'm talking to you. They must be real.[115]

The well-known medium Doris Stokes claims that she had her first encounter with 'spirits' when she was still a young child. Throughout her life she maintained contact with these 'spirits of the dead', held conversations with them, and conveyed their messages to large numbers of grateful and admiring people. Doris Stokes has documented many of her mediumistic experiences in books whose titles include *Voices In My Ear*, *A Host Of Voices*, and *Whispering Voices*.

Experiences which involve hearing the voices of what are claimed to be 'spirits', 'gods' or other supernatural entities appear not to be uncommon among human beings generally. It has even been suggested that experiences involving verbal contact with 'spirits' are quite common in young children. One reputable British psychiatrist has formed the opinion that from the age of 5 or 6 until puberty many children are 'clairaudient' and hear the voices of 'discarnate entities' which instruct them.[116] The renowned physician and thanatologist Dr Elisabeth Kübler-Ross believes that young children often have 'helping spirits' which take the form of their 'imaginary companions':

> Only a few of us who live in modern Western civilisation understand that benevolent 'helping spirits' and 'imaginary friends' are by no means projections of an imagination gone riot. The critically ill children in my care refer to these spirits as their 'playmates'. They are very real companions to them – guides and helpers at a time of isolation, loneliness, and suffering. Such companions are known by children everywhere. Only when children grow up in an unbelieving world, that tends to laugh at such follies, do they as a rule lose their ability to recognise these helpers.[117]

In many non-Western societies a range of techniques are routinely used to induce altered states of consciousness (ASCs) in which contact with various 'spirit beings' can occur. By such means a two-way communication may be established with the invisible presence of guardian spirits, angels, deceased ancestors and natural deities. A practice akin to mediumship is commonly employed by shamans (see below) as an integral part of their healing work. Indeed, the initiation, instruction and training of novice shamans is always conducted at least in part by 'spirits', some of which are likely to be those of the tribe's previously deceased shamans.

Trance Channelling

Whilst in a non-ordinary or altered state of consciousness (ASC) such as trance, some persons experience what they believe to be contact with non-physical 'entities' or 'beings' which are separate from and independent of themselves. Such beings usually appear in the guise of discarnate humans, non-human entities, or deities who supposedly inhabit higher planes of consciousness and who are said to be endowed with extraordinary intelligence and wisdom. The phenomenon which is now often referred to as 'channelling' is a contemporary form of mediumship in which such non-physical entities allegedly speak through the medium using his or her vocal apparatus. In some instances the 'higher being' communicates directly with the 'channel' (or medium) by means of spoken words which are heard privately and then reported to others:

> In non-ordinary states of consciousness . . . occasionally one can come into contact with an entity that appears to be entirely separate from and independent of one's own inner process. He or she offers a personal relationship and continues to play the role of guide, protector, teacher, or superior source of information. In the literature on psychic phenomena such figures are usually referred to as spirit guides . . . They communicate with their proteges through direct thought transfer or through other extrasensory means. Occasionally, they have human voices and send verbal messages.[118]

In the previous chapter a number of examples were given of prominent artistic individuals who claimed that the inspiration for some of their important creative works came in the form of 'dictation' received from invisible sources. John Milton, William Blake and Robert Schumann are notable examples of this process. In addition to such allegedly 'channelled' secular works there are others whose content is overtly spiritual in nature. Although the practice of utilising trance states in order to gain access to the spiritual guidance of higher beings is at least as old as the oracles of ancient Greece, much supposedly 'channelled' material has been dismissed as either fraudulent or superficial and trite. Nevertheless, a number of important and influential spiritual teachings are alleged to have originated directly from the voice of God, the angels, or various other elevated beings. Notable examples are the Ten Commandments, which God spoke directly to Moses, and the Koran, which was allegedly dictated to Mohammed by the archangel Gabriel.

An example of a hugely popular contemporary channelled work

is the book, *A Course in Miracles*.[119] The channel, Helen Schucman, was a professor of medical psychology at Columbia University's School of Physicians and Surgeons in New York. As a self-professed 'militant atheist' she very reluctantly received the text of this work from an uninvited inner voice which identified itself only as 'Christ'. Though at first worried that she might be developing a mental disorder Schucman eventually decided to simply write down all that she heard. Having no belief in God her ambivalence about the task was very great. She says that she resented the material she was taking down and felt strongly impelled to attack it and prove it wrong. The 500,000 word book which finally resulted from seven years of 'inner dictation' has been described as a restatement of the New Testament and a modern version of Gnostic Christianity. It has sold well over half a million copies and been translated into a dozen languages. When considered along with a number of other important spiritual works – which include the ancient Indian Vedas, the Koran (see above), the Book of Mormon, parts of the Bible, and several famous Tibetan Buddhist texts – it is clear that there are some allegedly 'channelled' works which have been of enormous spiritual significance both individually and culturally.

Shamanism

Anthropologists use the term 'shaman' to refer to the traditional healers who are found in many different cultures. Shamanic practices are very widespread and exist in various forms in all parts of the world including Siberia, China, Tibet, Japan, North and South America, Indonesia, South-East Asia, as well as amongst Australian Aborigines.[120] Known popularly as 'medicine men' or 'witch doctors', shamans are specifically empowered to do their healing work by virtue of their unique ability to communicate with 'spirits'. In every culture in which they are found shamans employ a wide range of socially sanctioned methods for entering altered states of consciousness in which they have immediate and concrete experiences with such spirits: they see and talk with them and implore their guidance and assistance in order to perform healing. The spirits with which the shaman communicates may take many guises and often appear in the form of animals, birds or other natural objects such as trees or clouds.

Those who become shamans usually do not choose this role for themselves but are instead 'called' to it by the spirits. Indeed, in some cultures self-made shamans are looked upon as inferior in power to those who have been so called. The call to become a shaman – which is reminiscent of the vocational call described by some Christians – often occurs during a period of illness (this is the so-called 'shamanic illness'). At this time visions, voices and various other unusual physical and emotional manifestations may occur as the neophyte shaman is initiated into the spirit world. This initiation usually involves an ascent to the 'Upper World' and a dialogue with the gods or spirits met there, and a descent to the 'Lower World' where conversations with spirits and the souls of dead shamans take place. By these means the spirits provide one part of the shaman's twofold course of instruction, the other part being provided by the older shamans of his tribe.[121]

An account provided by Black Elk, a highly respected American Indian holy man of the Oglala Sioux tribe, illustrates the way in which a person may be called by the spirits to become a shaman. The very first inkling of his future vocation occurred when Black Elk was only nine years old. One day, whilst he was eating, a voice came and said: 'It is time; now they are calling you.' The voice was so loud and clear that he believed it was real and decided to go where it wanted him to go. Shortly after this experience Black Elk became very sick, and the next day he had a vision in which two men carrying long spears spoke to him: 'Hurry! Come! Your Grandfathers are calling you!' For the next twelve days whilst he lay in a coma, Black Elk was taken to the 'spirit world' where many things were revealed to him. His experience culminated in a meeting with the six Grandfathers who instructed him. Many visions followed, including that of a great black stallion which sang to him:

> His voice was not loud, but it went all over the universe
> and filled it. There was nothing that did not hear, and it
> was more beautiful than anything can be. It was so beautiful
> that nothing anywhere could keep from dancing.[122]

Though he returned to the ordinary world following these experiences Black Elk was too young to understand them all and so, for several years, was afraid to speak of what he had seen and heard. Finally he revealed his vision and the instructions he had received when he sensed that the traditional ways of his tribe were being neglected. In this way he helped to nurture the spiritual strength of his people. At the end of his life Black Elk claimed that the words of the Grandfathers had always stayed with him in his heart: 'No words that I have ever heard with my ears were like the words I heard. I did not have to remember these things; they have remembered themselves all these years.'[123]

The newly-initiated shaman is often given specific guidance and instruction by his tutelary spirits in such matters as the type of instruments and materials he should use in order to be an effective healer. The following account illustrates a Siberian Samoyed shaman's instruction by means of visionary experiences which occurred during the three days of his initiatory sickness:

> Still preceded by his guides, the candidate then came to the Land of the Shamanesses, who strengthened his throat and his voice. He was then carried to the shores of the Nine Seas. In the middle of one of them was an island, and in the middle of the island a young birch tree rose to the sky. It was the Tree of the Lord of the Earth. Beside it grew nine herbs, the ancestors of all the plants on earth. The tree was surrounded by seas ... and, in the top of the tree [he] saw men of various nations. He heard voices: 'It has been decided that you shall have a drum (that is, the body of a drum) from the branches of this tree.' He began to fly with the birds of the seas. As he left the shore, the Lord of the tree called to him: 'My branch has just fallen; take it and make a drum of it that will serve you all your life.' The branch had three forks, and the Lord of the Tree bade him make three drums from it ... each drum being for a special ceremony ... Clasping the branch, the candidate was ready to resume his flight when again he heard a human voice, this time revealing to him the medicinal virtues of the seven plants and giving him certain instructions concerning the art of shamanizing.[124]

Shamanic practices are found amongst indigenous peoples throughout the world and, since the shaman's cosmos is filled with spirits, one of his important roles is to help others communicate with them. Anthropological research has shown that in many traditional societies such communing with 'spirits' does indeed play a major role in the ritual life of the community. One researcher found that it was an accepted practice in 62% of a world-wide sample of 488 societies studied.[125]

It is important to note that shamanic beliefs and practices such as those described above are no longer confined to traditional or pre-technological societies. During the past few decades there has been a burgeoning of interest in shamanism among Western anthropologists and, in addition, many lay-persons have experimented with activities based on traditional shamanic ceremonies and rituals in their quest for spiritual fulfilment. The growing acceptance of shamanism as a valid, culturally-relevant approach to spirituality and healing is particularly evident among many holistic health care practitioners, as well as some mental health professionals. As an example, in a recent innovative development a range of shamanic techniques have been successfully employed in treating people in a community mental health centre. Interestingly, approximately two-thirds of the clients with long histories of troublesome auditory hallucinations have reported experiencing immediate relief as a result.[126]

Conclusion

This chapter has shown that genuinely spiritual inner voice experiences have affected the lives of countless individuals and shaped the beliefs of large social groups and entire religious movements. There is little doubt that they have been a powerful influence for good throughout the world. So important have these phenomena been in human life generally that the Biblical story of Adam and Eve (even if it is allegorical) tells that one of the first experiences human beings had at the very beginning of creation was to hear the voice of God speaking in the Garden of Eden! It is interesting to reflect on the fact that several of the world's major religions (Christianity, Judaism and Islam) had their origins in spiritual voice experiences and that the lives of vast numbers of people have been touched in one way or another as a result. Even those who choose not to follow the precepts of the Christian faith cannot avoid its indirect influence since they, too, must live in a society whose moral, ethical and legal codes are largely based on values derived from the Ten Commandments and other imperatives given to humankind by means of supernatural voices. The same is true in Islamic, Jewish and other cultures.

In contemporary Western societies spirituality remains one of the very few areas in which people may have voice experiences without necessarily being viewed as mentally disturbed. Nevertheless, it is also common for people who have a psychiatric diagnosis to hear voices which, for a time at least, they believe have a supernatural origin. This fact raises an extremely important question: how is it possible to differentiate true spiritual voice experiences from those which come from other sources and which have an altogether different significance? As this chapter has shown, the guiding lights of the early Church were well aware of the possibility of deception and were consequently much concerned with this issue. Undoubtedly the easiest way to deal with this challenging problem is to lump all voice experiences together, label them as symptoms of mental disorder, and deny that any of them have any value. While this approach is appealingly simple it involves the risk of 'throwing out the baby with the bathwater'. The medieval saints went to very great lengths to address these issues. At the same time as wishing to protect people from being led astray they were also able to acknowledge the precious value of *true* spiritual experience. One of the greatest legacies of their profound wisdom is the practical guidelines they provided for differentiating between voice experiences that are truly spiritual and those that only appear to be so. Details of these guidelines for discernment can be found in Chapter Seven together with a discussion of another phenomenon often associated with apparently supernatural voices: the realm of spirits.

With the resurgence of interest in spirituality that is reflected both in the revival of esoteric practices of mainstream religions and the huge popularity of experiential approaches such as spiritualism, channelling and shamanism it seems certain that transcendent inner voices will remain an important source of spiritual nourishment and healing in our increasingly secular modern world.

Chapter Three

VOICES AND MENTAL ILLNESS

> *We cannot ignore the fact that a hallucinatory disposition is, to
> some extent, present in every psyche, and that schizophrenia,
> as well as other conditions, merely makes it manifest.*
>
> – Eugen Bleuler[127]

Many people consider the experience of hearing voices to be an
unequivocal symptom of severe mental illness.* In light of the
evidence presented in the previous two chapters which showed that
there are numerous circumstances in which people who are un-
questionably mentally healthy can have voice experiences of various
kinds, this view is clearly excessively narrow and unwarranted.
Nevertheless, voices can and often do occur as either a prominent
or a minor feature of a wide range of mental disorders. This chapter
provides an overview of some of these disorders together with a
description of the types of voice experiences which may occur in
association with them.

Voices and Sensory Deception

Before considering these disorders in more detail it is worthwhile
reflecting briefly on the history of how hearing voices came to be
seen as an indicator of mental illness. As was pointed out in Chapter
Two, during the Middle Ages the way people throughout Europe

---

* The term 'mental illness' is used here in deference to the fact that
  currently it is widely used and accepted. Nevertheless, the author has
  grave reservations regarding the appropriateness of referring to mental
  disorders or disturbances as 'illnesses'. Many others have voiced similar
  concerns. For an articulate and well-informed discussion of this issue
  see psychiatry professor Thomas Szasz's profound and important book,
  The Myth of Mental Illness (New York: Harper and Row, 1961).

experienced the world was strongly influenced by religious teachings and beliefs. Consequently, anyone who saw or heard things related to non-physical causes was simply considered to have had a vision or received a revelation from some supernatural source, be it good or evil. Similar views still prevail in many non-Western societies where highly tolerant attitudes often exist toward experiences which involve seeing or hearing things not physically present. A range of possible interpretations are given to such experiences, many of which are considered benign and of no particular consequence, whilst others are looked upon as highly desirable in certain circumstances.[128] As was the case in medieval Europe, in non-Western societies the presence of mental illness is generally inferred on the basis of a person's aberrant, inappropriate or socially unacceptable *behaviour* rather than according to any particular kind of perceptual experience they may have. This implies that so long as a person's behaviour does not exceed the limits of socially-accepted norms and expectations they might hear voices (or have visions) and still be considered quite normal.[129]

Rather ironically it appears that the great sixteenth-century Spanish mystic, St Teresa of Avila, whose own spiritual life was immeasurably enriched by supernatural voices ('locutions'), may have contributed to the gradually changing way in which experiences involving voices and visions were viewed by Europeans.[130] In an effort to protect the nuns in her abbey from the machinations of the Inquisition (which had the power to condemn to death anyone convicted of practising witchcraft, a fate which eventually befell Joan of Arc), Teresa argued that certain of their revelationary and visionary experiences may have been due to natural, rather than supernatural, causes. Among these she identified melancholy, a weak imagination, drowsiness, and sleep or sleep-like states. Whilst this pronouncement undoubtedly helped save many people from torture or execution at the stake it introduced a notion which was to have very far-reaching consequences. It had been St Teresa's intention to maintain a distinction between those voices and visions which were related to supernatural causes and those which were not, but with the increasing secularisation of society this distinction was gradually lost. In time, *all* such experiences began to be looked upon as abnormal and anyone who admitted to having them was automatically considered to be in need of treatment.

Voices as Hallucinations

The Oxford English Dictionary explains that, when it entered the English language in 1652, the first meanings of the word 'hallucination' (derived from the Latin *alucinari*, 'to wander in mind') were 'to be deceived, suffer illusion, entertain false notions, blunder, mistake'. By the early nineteenth-century the first scientific attempts were being made to understand and classify various kinds of unusual perceptual experience and in 1832 the French physician Jean Esquirol used the word hallucination in the way that is still accepted by modern psychologists and psychiatrists. In his influential work, *Mental Maladies: A Treatise on Insanity*, Esquirol proclaimed:

> A person is said to labor under a hallucination . . . who has a thorough conviction of the perception of a sensation, when no external object, suited to excite this sensation, has impressed the senses.[131]

Most contemporary definitions are derived from the one first proposed by Esquirol. Thus, in the American Psychiatric Association's 1994 Glossary of Technical Terms an hallucination is defined as: 'A sensory perception that has the compelling sense of reality of a true perception but that occurs without external stimulation of the relevant sensory organ.'[132] According to this definition the experience of hearing voices would be classed as a 'verbal auditory hallucination'. As described below, such phenomena are a frequent accompaniment of many types of mental disorder.

For convenience mental disorders are often classified into one of two broad categories. Those associated with an identifiable physical cause affecting the brain and nervous system make up one group, the so-called *organic mental disorders*. Those which do not have an identifiable physical cause and for which non-physical (i.e. psychological, social, spiritual) factors play a more significant causal role make up the other group and are referred to as *functional mental disorders*. As discussed below, hallucinations of various kinds may be associated with disorders belonging to both of these two groups.

Organic Mental Disorders

There are a wide range of medical disorders and conditions which can either directly or indirectly interfere with or impair the functioning of the brain and which may, as a consequence, lead to the development of various kinds of organic mental disorder. In many cases the causative factors can be readily identified by means of physical examinations and various laboratory tests. It is also possible that some people who develop a psychiatric disorder may have an *undetected* physical illness or condition which has directly contributed to their disturbed mental state. This is probably not an uncommon occurrence. For example, in one study in which 658 psychiatric outpatients were given a thorough medical and biochemical examination, 9.1% were found to have a physical condition which contributed to their psychiatric disorder.[133] It is noteworthy that in almost half of these cases neither the person concerned nor their treating physician were aware of the illness until the examinations were done.

The following are among the most significant of the many organic mental disorders in which hallucinations may occur as a prominent feature:

1 *Psychotic Disorders related to Organic Causes*

A psychotic disorder involves a state of extreme mental and emotional disturbance in which the affected person experiences a number of the following: fixed false beliefs ('delusions'); unshared sensory perceptions ('hallucinations'); markedly illogical or disorganised thinking ('thought disorder'); and labile or inappropriate emotions. As a result of these experiences the person may be said to be 'out of touch with reality' (i.e. consensual reality) to a greater or lesser degree.

Compromised brain functioning sometimes leads to the development of a psychotic state in which hallucinations of various kinds may be a prominent feature, although these are more often visual than auditory. Medical conditions associated with psychosis can include: infections such as viral encephalitis (Herpes, HIV), meningitis (bacterial or viral), and syphilis; exogenous toxins such as amphetamines, cocaine, hallucinogens (LSD, PCP, mescaline), steroids, barbiturates (intoxication or withdrawal), heavy metals, and anticholinergic drugs; alcohol withdrawal states (hallucinosis and delirium tremens); endocrine imbalances associated with adrenal, thyroid and parathyroid disorder; metabolic disorders such as porphyria, electrolyte imbalances, end-stage kidney or liver failure; space-occupying lesions such as subdural haematoma and brain abscesses; nutritional deficiencies including niacin and thiamine; vascular abnormalities such as collagen disorders, aneurysm and intracranial haemorrhage; head trauma of various kinds (commonly from right-sided injury); cerebral hypoxia secondary to decreased cardiac or respiratory output or blood loss; and epilepsy, most notably involving the temporal lobe.[134]

2 *Delirium (Acute Organic Brain Syndrome)*

Delirium is a relatively common mental disorder characterised by a generalised though transient disturbance of consciousness. Its main features include disorientation for time, place, and person, and impaired thinking, comprehension, memory, perception, and attention. A delirium can occur as a result of impairment of normal brain functioning due to a range of medical conditions and illnesses. These may include: cerebral and systemic infections; alcohol and drug intoxication or withdrawal; metabolic disturbances; head injury; and intracranial tumour. Hallucinations are quite common in delirious states though they are usually fleeting in nature and almost invariably visual rather than auditory.[135]

3 *Drug Intoxication and Withdrawal*

The hallucinations induced by psychoactive drugs are predominantly visual in nature. If auditory hallucinations do occur they tend to be elemental or unformed (e.g. indistinct noises), although more complex experiences, including voices, do sometimes occur. For example, chronic cocaine abuse can result in the development of a 'cocaine psychosis', which is a subacute delirious state characterised by auditory hallucinations with persecutory content.[136] Ingestion of large quantities of marijuana or potent hashish can also precipitate an acute psychotic state in which persecutory voices may be a prominent feature. Following the use of an hallucinogenic drug such as LSD some people may later re-experience one or more of the perceptual experiences that occurred whilst they were under the influence of the drug. These experiences (sometimes known as 'flashbacks') may include auditory hallucinations of sounds or voices. Though 'flashbacks' usually only last for a few seconds cases have been reported in which they have occurred throughout the day for years on end.[137] Whilst withdrawing from alcohol or sedative and hypnotic drugs some people develop an abstinence syndrome or withdrawal reaction with delirious features. Vivid hallucinations, whether visual, auditory, or tactile are a common feature of this withdrawal delirium. Delirium tremens (commonly known as 'DTs' or 'the horrors') is a relatively uncommon disorder which occurs during or following the abrupt cessation of drinking in a small proportion of chronic alcoholic persons. This delirious state is characterised by primarily visual and tactile hallucinations, though auditory hallucinations can also occur. The hallucinations which accompany alcohol withdrawal are transitory, usually lasting for only a few days.[138]

4 *Organic Hallucinosis*

Organic hallucinosis is a mental disorder directly attributed to some clearly defined organic factor (e.g. chronic alcohol or hallucinogen abuse) in which recurrent or persistent hallucinations are the predominant or *only* symptom. The hallucinations may occur in one or more sensory modalities although auditory hallucinations appear to be the most common type. Alcoholic hallucinosis is a relatively rare condition characterised by mainly auditory hallucinations which persist following withdrawal from alcohol in a person who is no longer drinking. The affected person typically hears threatening, criticising, or insulting voices which speak about him or her in the third person.[139] Sometimes the voices are benign and have little effect on the person's behaviour. The auditory hallucinations in some cases of hallucinosis seem to begin as elementary sounds which then evolve into the more complex experience of distinct voices:

> Early on, the patient becomes aware of formless acoustic perceptions, such as crackling, knocking or roaring noises, the ringing of bells, or sibilant sounds like a half-heard whisper. Gradually these noises take on more form and become articulate. He hears the voices of friends and enemies, accusing him of drinking, of sex offences, of real or imaginary misdeeds in his past life.[140]

A state of alcoholic hallucinosis may be as brief as a few hours or days or it may persist for several months. In some cases it may become chronic. (Some authorities have suggested that in those cases in which the hallucinatory voices do become permanent the affected person may have an underlying schizophrenic-type disorder which has been unmasked by long-term alcohol abuse. There continues to be considerable controversy regarding this particular view.)

Functional Mental Disorders

In contrast to the organic disorders described above there is no known physical cause to account for the mental disorders which are classified as functional. It is probable that a complex interplay of emotional, psychological, social, and spiritual factors contribute to the causation of these disturbances. It is also possible that biological factors sometimes play a role (e.g. in some cases there may be some kind of genetic predisposition). The hallucinations which occur in association with functional disorders are often auditory, and voices can occur as a prominent feature in a number of these disorders. Before discussing functional disorders generally it is worth noting that the experience of hearing voices has come to be particularly associated with schizophrenia in the minds of many people, including many mental health professionals. As a consequence, it is quite likely that some people who are hearing voices as part of a functional mental disorder may be *inappropriately* given a diagnosis of schizophrenia when one of the other diagnoses listed below may actually be more apt.

The following are the main functional mental disorders in which auditory hallucinations may occur as a prominent feature:

1 *Psychotic Depression*

Severe depression is sometimes accompanied by hallucinations which take the form of voices. The voices, which are usually transient and limited to single words or short phrases, are generally heard to say things consistent with the person's depressed mood. Thus, a psychotically depressed person may hear voices which are derisive and humiliating, and which berate him or her for sundry shortcomings, failures, and sins, whether these be real or imagined. A depressed person may be accused of various sexual or other misdemeanours and they might be ordered by the voices to perform expiatory acts, possibly even including acts of self-mutilation or even suicide.[141] Although psychotic depression is considered to be the most severe form of depression it is not uncommon. Some studies suggest that as many as one quarter of all depressed persons may be suffering from psychotic depression.[142]

2 Manic Episode and Bipolar Disorder

A manic episode – which can occur on its own or in combination with one or more episodes of depression as part of Bipolar Disorder (formerly known as 'Manic Depression') – involves a distinct period of abnormally and persistently elevated, expansive, or irritable mood. Though it is often believed that relatively few manic individuals hear voices this may not actually be the case. In one study, for example, 47% of such persons reported auditory hallucinations.[143] The auditory hallucinations which occur in manic episodes usually involve hearing voices which speak directly to the person and whose content is congruent with their abnormally elevated mood. Thus, for example, God's voice may be heard explaining the person's special mission in life, or the voices may say things like 'Go to the palace! You are the king!'[144] Manic persons have also reported experiences such as hearing the hallelujah chorus from Handel's 'Messiah' or holding conversations with a dead daughter.[145]

3 Schizophrenia

A person may be given a diagnosis of schizophrenia if they experience a psychosis characterised by: delusions which seem to be 'bizarre' or totally implausible; hallucinations, especially in the form of voices; markedly illogical or disorganised thinking; emotional disturbances including inappropriate, blunted or flattened affect; and grossly disorganised or catatonic behaviour. The duration of these symptoms is particularly important since schizophrenia is currently defined as a disturbance which lasts for at least six months, during which time psychotic symptoms such as delusions and hallucinations must have been present for at least one month (less if treated).[146] For a diagnosis of schizophrenia to be made it must be established that the disturbance is *not* due to alcohol or drug use, physical illness, or a mood disorder such as mania or depression. If the person's symptoms have lasted more than one day but less than a month they may be diagnosed as having a *Brief Psychotic Disorder* rather than schizophrenia. If the psychosis involves a mixture of prominent mood symptoms (such as mania or depression) and schizophrenia symptoms, the diagnosis of *Schizoaffective Disorder* may be made.

Auditory hallucinations in the form of voices have long been considered one of the most characteristic symptoms of schizophrenia. Indeed, it has been estimated that about 70% of people with this diagnosis hear voices of some kind.[147] The Diagnostic and Statistical Manual of Mental Disorders (DSM-IV), which lists the American Psychiatric Association's official diagnostic criteria for schizophrenia, makes no distinction as to whether the voices are heard inside the head or as coming from outside.[148] The person hearing such voices perceives them to be distinct from his or her own thoughts and, though their content can be quite variable, often experiences them as being pejorative or threatening. Certain types of voices, such as two or more voices conversing with one another, or voices which keep up a running commentary on the person's thoughts or behaviour, are considered to be particularly characteristic of schizophrenia and are often included among the list of so-called 'First Rank Symptoms' devised by Kurt Schneider. In fact, the presence of these symptoms alone would be sufficient to convince many psychiatrists that it was appropriate to make a diagnosis of schizophrenia. It is important to note that for hallucinations (auditory or otherwise) to be considered symptoms of schizophrenia they must be distinguished from sensory experiences which might occur to *any* person in dreams or when falling asleep or waking up (such normal 'hypnagogic' and 'hypnopompic' experiences were described in Chapter One). Furthermore, isolated experiences of hearing one's name called, or certain unusual sensory experiences which might occur in a religious or spiritual context in some cultures, are also not necessarily indicative of schizophrenia.

Note: Because schizophrenia is considered to be the most common major mental disorder and because the experience of hearing voices is so often associated with it the whole of Chapter Four will be devoted to a detailed discussion of the voices of schizophrenia.

4 *Multiple Personality Disorder (also called 'Dissociative Identity Disorder')*

The characteristic feature of Multiple Personality Disorder (MPD) is the existence within a person of two or more distinct personalities or personality states, each of which is able to take control of the person's behaviour.[149] Although MPD has long been considered an extremely rare syndrome there is growing evidence that it might not be as uncommon as was once thought. One psychiatrist who is an authority on MPD has estimated that anywhere between 1 in 50 and 1 in 10,000 persons in urban North America might be affected by this syndrome, and that between 2% and 5% of all psychiatric inpatients might have full, classical MPD.[150] In the vast majority of cases of MPD severe and prolonged early childhood sexual or physical abuse is believed to be the principal causative factor.

The various personalities (so-called 'alters') that coexist within a person with MPD often have a degree of awareness of some or all of the others and may experience them as friends, companions or adversaries. Frequently, one or more of the personalities has the experience of hearing the voice(s) of one or more of the other alter personalities. This sometimes occurs as a precursor to an alter personality assuming executive control:

> People with multiple personality disorder often hear the voice of an 'alter' for weeks before it first acquires power to enter the body at will. They perceive the alter's voice as coming from *inside their head* ... Even after the alter gains the ability to take command, some MPD sufferers can hear it speaking while it is not in the body, but 'nearby'. Alters usually lack the threatening quality of schizophrenic voices or the grandiose tone of manic voices.[151]

In one study of the experiences of people with MPD, 64% said they had heard voices.[152] In another study hearing voices was the most commonly reported symptom of all.[153] A very wide range of variation exists in the nature and quality of these voices:

> It is a general rule of thumb that MPD voices tend to come from inside the head ... [they] may be commanding and persecutory and may order the patient to harm herself or others. Alternatively, they may be soothing and reassuring. The two types of voices may discuss the patient, referring

to her in the third person. Usually the MPD patient does not have a thought disorder and describes the voices in a lucid manner. The content of the voices' statements is usually not bizarre and 'crazy', though it may be.[154]

Although it has been formally recognised by the American Psychiatric Association as a bona fide mental disorder since 1980 considerable controversy nevertheless continues to surround MPD. Some authorities believe that it is a drastically *under*-diagnosed condition and that some people who have been given a diagnosis of schizophrenia may actually have unrecognised MPD. On the other hand, however, there are those who feel that it has been vastly *over*-diagnosed and that it is a rare condition (if indeed it exists at all).

Note: A detailed discussion of the voices of MPD and some of the other controversial issues surrounding this extraordinary condition can be can be found in Chapter Five.

5 *Post-Traumatic Stress Disorder (PTSD)*

Post-Traumatic Stress Disorder (PTSD) is a syndrome which some people may develop as a consequence of having been exposed to an extremely traumatic stressor sufficient to provoke the experience of intense fear, helplessness or horror. The characteristic symptoms of PTSD involve re-experiencing the traumatic event (e.g. intrusive dreams, 'flashbacks'), avoidance of stimuli associated with the original event, a numbing of general emotional responsiveness, and increased arousal.[155] Some people may re-experience the original traumatic event via the medium of auditory hallucinations. For example, a recent research study found that 27% of a group of survivors of childhood incest heard voices later in life.[156] Some combat veterans with PTSD also report hearing persistent voices, usually of a depressive nature and involving cries for help or conversations concerning battle.[157] In some cases of combat-related PTSD the voices have been directly related to a specific and particularly distressing occurrence, as the following example illustrates:

> Mr. B, a 55 year old Hispanic veteran, had fought for 6 months in the Korean war when he was 18 years old . . . his auditory hallucinations and other symptoms focused on one

specific event: shooting a young North Korean soldier who was wounded. Auditory hallucinations involving a voice, ascribed to the Korean, that berated the patient and told him to commit suicide began about one week later and had continued ever since. The voice was perceived as coming from the patient's environment, not within his head.[158]

It has recently been recognised that some people who have been severely psychotic may be sufficiently traumatised by the experience of psychosis and/or subsequent enforced hospitalisation and treatment that they develop a Post-Traumatic Stress Disorder.[159] Since voices can occur as a prominent feature of PTSD it is possible that some people whose persistent auditory hallucinations have been attributed to a psychotic disorder such as schizophrenia may actually be continuing to hear voices as part of a post-psychotic PTSD.

6 *Post-partum Psychosis*

Post-partum disorders involve a range of disturbances which women can develop in the period shortly after giving birth. They include affective and organic-like mental disorders and functional psychoses, with depression being the most common ('baby blues'). Disturbances which involve psychotic manifestations such as hallucinations have often been described as rare, only occurring in about 1 or 2 out of every 1000 deliveries.[160] However, in one study of 100 women with a range of post-partum disorders, 12 appeared to have conversion hallucinations.[161] (see below) The symptoms of post-partum disorders are centred on the woman's feelings about the newborn baby and her role as a mother. A mother who hallucinates during a post-partum psychotic disturbance may hear voices telling her to kill her baby, or she may hear accusatory voices regarding her lack of fitness to be a mother. On the other hand, some women simply hear their baby crying.

7 *Conversion Disorder ('Hysteria')*

Conversion disorders involve an alteration or loss of physical functioning which suggest a physical disorder but which have no physiological cause and are actually the expression of some underlying psychological conflict or need. Conversion symptoms usually develop in the context of extreme psychological distress and often appear quite suddenly. Although the most common manifestations are deafness, blindness, and paralysis a number of researchers have shown that hallucinations can occur as conversion symptoms.[162] An example of this is the case of a young Indian girl whose principal complaint was a disturbing voice which began when she was required to change classes at school. This change caused her great distress because she would have to be with strangers and in place of her favourite teacher she would have one who was more strict. After several days of severe emotional turmoil the girl suddenly began to hear a voice:

> As soon as she entered the door of her new class she began hearing a voice which said, 'Come, come, don't be in the class'. Interestingly, though her mother tongue is Kannada, the voice spoke in English – the medium of instruction in her school. K. felt afraid but entered the class nevertheless. The voice seemed to emanate from near the door, but nobody was to be seen there ... [it] continued incessantly right through the day, repeating its stereotyped message like a gramophone needle stuck in a groove ... The voice was that of a young lady, heard in clear consciousness with K. having no ability to influence or modify it in any way. She had no idea as to whom the voice could have belonged or why it should torment her so. The voice disappeared the moment she left the class.[163]

Each time this girl attended the class over the next week she heard the same voice which began as she entered the classroom. The voice persisted with its stereotyped message as long as she remained in the class but disappeared the instant she left. When she was eventually put back into her original class the voice stopped permanently. Some authorities have suggested that among Asian women (especially teenagers), the most common cause of hallucinatory experiences is not in fact schizophrenia but hysterical conversion.[164]

Conclusion

Hearing voices is an experience which occurs in association with many mental disorders. However, since all of these disorders can involve a wide range of possible symptomatic manifestations which are influenced by a complex interplay of many internal and external factors, it is hardly surprising to find that voices, if and when they occur, also vary considerably according to the personal characteristics of the hearer and the specific details of his or her psychological, social, spiritual, and biological circumstances. As a consequence, voice experiences may vary greatly from one person to another even though they have the *same* psychiatric diagnosis. The fact that recent research has failed to find a close connection between the qualitative characteristics of people's voice hearing experiences and their psychiatric diagnosis lends considerable support to the notion that, even when it occurs in association with a particular psychiatric disorder, hearing voices is always a highly individualised experience.[165]

Many people with a psychiatric disorder hear voices which are frightening, intrusive and disturbing in various ways. In addition to the immediate impact of these voices the stigma that is associated with actually hearing them often adds to the diagnosed person's burden. For this reason many people choose to conceal the existence of their voices from others, perhaps even from mental health professionals. Because there has for a very long time been a lack of truly effective assistance (whether pharmacological or psychotherapeutic) many diagnosed persons have suffered greatly as a result of persistent and disturbing voices. Fortunately during the past decade or so there has been renewed interest in gaining a better understanding of voice hearing experiences and providing more helpful kinds of support. One of the most important recent developments has been the recognition that there are a wide range of practical strategies which may help people to prevent or ameliorate disturbing voices (many of these are described in detail in Chapter Eight). The advent of pragmatic approaches such as these has meant that many people are now being empowered – often for the very first time – to take control of their disturbing voice experiences.

Although they often cause significant distress it is important to be aware that not all voices which occur in the context of mental disorder are necessarily experienced as negative. It is a fact that many people find their voices to be positive or helpful in some way and that many hear a *mixture* of both positive and negative voices. It is interesting to note, furthermore, that the early pioneers of psychiatry were inclined to view voices rather differently to the way they are usually seen today. For example, Sigmund Freud believed that hallucinatory voices often served as restitutive symptoms. In other words, he saw them as the diagnosed person's (unconscious) attempt to re-establish an emotional connection to a valued person or persons following the loss of that connection in the ordinary social world.[166] Many others who have followed this line of thinking have emphasised the possible adaptive value of voices. For example, Professor Silvano Arieti has suggested that in some cases they may be manifestations of a vital defensive manoeuvre and that the transformation of inner emotional conflicts into hallucinatory symptoms which refer to the external world is often psychologically advantageous to the diagnosed person.[167] Views such as these emphasise the social and psychological aspects of voice experiences and consider them to be at least as pertinent – if not more so – than the biological aspects. For a number of complex reasons such ideas have now largely fallen out of favour.

Because a great deal can be learnt both theoretically (in terms of throwing light on how and why voices occur) and practically (fostering greater empathic understanding and gaining insight into what can be done to provide more effective help) the following two chapters will be devoted to a discussion of the voice experiences which occur in association with schizophrenia and multiple personality disorder.

Chapter Four
THE VOICES OF SCHIZOPHRENIA

For the purpose of demonstrating clearly that the essence of the hallucinatory process lies in the psyche organ no other disease is as well suited as schizophrenia. For, aside from many other reasons, hallucinations do not express sensory material but thoughts, feelings, and drives.

– Eugen Bleuler[168]

In many people's minds the experience of hearing voices is inextricably linked with schizophrenia. The fact that voice experiences are *not* confined to this or any other kind of 'mental illness' has now been amply demonstrated. Nevertheless, because schizophrenia is so commonly diagnosed (it is often said to be a condition that affects between 1% and 2% of the entire human population), and since voice experiences of various kinds *are* indeed extremely common among people given this diagnosis, particular attention will be devoted to it. The fact that many people who live with schizophrenia suffer tremendously as a result of disturbing voices in itself justifies a closer scrutiny of their experiences since developing a better understanding of them may enhance the ability of helpers and other concerned persons to empathise and thus provide better and more effective help and support. On a broader level this undertaking raises many questions of great theoretical and practical importance regarding the nature of schizophrenia and will hopefully contribute to the extremely important task of improving our understanding of this most mysterious and enigmatic state of mind.

Before proceeding it is important to be aware that there are a number of potential sources of misunderstanding and confusion which can impede straightforward discussion of this topic. For one thing, there is an unfortunately common tendency to assume that once a person has been given a diagnosis of schizophrenia (or any

other psychiatric diagnosis for that matter) *everything* they experience or do – especially if it seems a bit odd or unusual – must be
a direct manifestation of their mental condition. It should be
remembered, however, that in addition to hearing voices which may
be specifically related to schizophrenia, people with this diagnosis
might also have the same kinds of voice experiences that *all* human
beings are prone to. As was described in previous chapters, voices
can occur in connection with sleep, dreams, spirituality, bereavement, stress, extreme isolation, sensory deprivation, childhood
abuse, post-traumatic stress disorder (PTSD) and a range of other
circumstances. It is possible, therefore, that some of a diagnosed
person's voice experiences might be related to factors quite apart
from schizophrenia. This possibility should not be overlooked by
people living with schizophrenia nor by those involved in providing
assessment, treatment and care.

It should also be pointed out that there are many highly
regarded authorities who question the traditional psychiatric view
linking voices with schizophrenia.[169] Some have suggested that the
apparent association may come about not because voices are one of
the most common symptoms of schizophrenia, but because people
who hear voices of *any* kind are highly likely to be given this
particular diagnosis. This possibility was dramatically demonstrated
in 1973 by David Rosenhan, a Stanford University psychologist
who conducted an experiment which highlighted the extent to which
the experience of hearing voices may be taken at face value as a
symptom of schizophrenia by mental health professionals.[170]
Rosenhan arranged for a number of 'normal' mentally healthy
volunteers to attend the admissions offices of several psychiatric
hospitals with the sole complaint that they had been hearing voices.
When asked what the voices said they replied that they were often
unclear but seemed to be saying 'empty', 'hollow' and 'thud'. The
voices were described as being unfamiliar and of the same sex as
the volunteer. Despite the fact that voices were the *only* symptom
complained of, all the volunteers were admitted as in-patients and
all but one were given a diagnosis of schizophrenia (the exception,
who was diagnosed manic-depressive, had gained admission to the
only private psychiatric hospital approached for the experiment).
Immediately after admission all of the volunteers ceased simulating
any symptoms of abnormality (including voices) and from then on
behaved completely normally. They were nevertheless hospitalised

for periods ranging from 7 to 52 days (the average being 19 days) and prescribed a variety of psychotropic medications. The fact that the volunteers were actually mentally normal was never detected by the hospital staff although the other patients on the wards were often quite suspicious of them. All the pseudo-patients were discharged with the diagnosis 'schizophrenia in remission', which led Rosenhan to comment on the tendency of diagnostic labels to stick to people once they have been attached. The complex issues raised by this thought-provoking experiment should be borne in mind when reading the material that follows.

The Experience of Hearing Voices

Since Professor Eugen Bleuler introduced the concept of schizophrenia to psychiatry in 1911 the experience of hearing voices has always been seen as one of the most characteristic symptoms of this disorder. Indeed, it has been estimated that about 70% of people with a diagnosis of schizophrenia hear voices of some kind.* Despite clear evidence that voices can occur in conjunction with many types of mental disorder and that healthy 'normal' people can also experience them, in everyday clinical practice the presence of 'verbal auditory hallucinations' often strongly influences what psychiatric diagnosis a person will be given (as Rosenhan's experiment made clear). Many mental health professionals still consider voices to be a pathognomonic symptom of schizophrenia. Thus, as one influential textbook states:

> Auditory hallucinations in the form of voices are the commonest schizophrenic symptom and are often diagnostic of the condition ... the hallucinatory voice is characteristically schizophrenic, so that if in a state of clear consciousness a patient hears well-organised voices consisting of more than one sentence he should be diagnosed as

---

* It appears that even deaf people with a diagnosis of schizophrenia may 'hear' voices! Thus, in a study of twelve prelingually profoundly deaf persons, ten were found to have had experiences analogous to auditory hallucinations. In one case the man concerned could see the arms and hands of a person finger spelling and signing to him (see Critchley et al., 1981).

suffering from schizophrenia unless it can be proved otherwise. Or to put it in another way, continuous auditory hallucinosis in the absence of coarse brain disease is due to schizophrenia.[171]

A very wide range of experiences may be associated with the voices. Thus, people living with schizophrenia may hear blowing, rustling, humming, rattling, shooting, thundering, music, crying, laughing, whispering and talking.[172] The voices heard can also vary enormously in terms of their character and content:

> They converse, threaten, curse, criticise, consult, often in short sentences. They admonish, console, mock, command, or sometimes simply announce everything that's happening. They yell, whine, sneer, and vary from the slightest whisper to a thunderous shout. Often the voices take on some special peculiarity, such as speaking very slowly, scanning, rhyming, or in rhythms, or even in foreign languages. There may be one particular voice, more often a few voices, and occasionally many ... they are recognised as gods, angels, devils, enemies, or a particular person or relative. Or occasionally they are ascribed to some kind of apparatus ... [173]

Hallucinatory experiences which involve one or more of the diagnosed person's other senses (i.e. sight, touch, taste or smell) sometimes occur in conjunction with voices.* The voices themselves are sometimes accompanied by non-verbal sounds such as music, laughter, crying, animal noises, and so on. Such sounds may lend emphasis and verisimilitude to what the voices say. For example, when John Perceval heard the sounds of a choir of angels his hopes of salvation were raised, but later, when the heavenly voice which accused him of disobedience to the faith was accompanied by 'the clanking of iron, and the breathing of great

---

* Interestingly, in non-Western cultures people with a diagnosis of schizophrenia tend to experience *visual* hallucinations more often than auditory ones. It seems that in Western society auditory hallucinations may have only become the predominant type during the course of the last century (see Slade and Bentall, 1988).

forge bellows, and the force of flames', he was sure he had been condemned into hell.[174]

The Onset of the Voices

The voices can begin in a number of different ways. Sometimes they are almost imperceptible at first, perhaps originating in the person's own thoughts which are gradually transformed into vague whispers that eventually become louder and more distinct. One person, for example, felt his voice experiences had involved day dreams which progressed to dominant thoughts and then finally to a voice. Voices may occasionally begin in a person's dreams:

> In some cases the hallucinations slip into the patient's consciousness almost entirely unnoticed. Certain thoughts continue to become more vivid till they assume a sensory character; or it all starts with a very gentle, vague whisper which was at first scarcely noticed. A patient feels her thoughts dividing. 'It began to talk loudly as if it were inside the brain.' In rare cases, the hallucinations first appear as the ordinary dream; then they appear in the hypnagogic state; then finally in the full waking state.[175]

One woman who first started hearing 'ghostly voices' coming from her closet when she was only eight years old said about them: 'I do not know when it was that I first started hearing voices – they were just there and I think they had probably been going on for some time before I was consciously aware of them.'[176] Another person's experience exemplified the very gradual onset of voices:

> It began gradually while I was spending a lot of time alone in my apartment. At first it was just a feeling that something was watching me, like a presence. Then I'd see something moving out of the corner of my eye, but when I'd look directly there would be nothing there. The voices began as a kind of background chatter too soft to make out exactly, like gurgles in a stream. I became convinced that someone was in my apartment, so I'd search from room to room and find no one. It got really scary when I heard something whispering my name over and over ... After a couple of days of this I started to hear whole conversations among

individual voices: a woman, a man, then another woman, mostly laughing and poking fun at me. Sometimes they seemed good-natured, but at other times they would curse and insult me.[177]

In the beginning some people may have to consciously work at actually hearing, and then trying to understand, what the voices are saying:

At first I'd had to strain just to hear or understand them. They were soft and working with some pretty tricky codes. Snap-crackle-pops, the sound of the wind with blinking lights and horns for punctuation. I broke the code and somehow was able to internalise it to the point where it was just like hearing words. In the beginning it seemed mostly nonsense, but as things went along they made more and more sense. Once you hear the voices, you realise they've always been there. It's just a matter of being tuned to them.[178]

The voices sometimes begin quite abruptly. In such cases the hearer may be struck right from the start by an audible voice which has a powerful emotional impact. The following example provides a graphic illustration of this kind of startling experience:

One day I went to reconnoitre in New York City's East Side. Being a stranger I was surprised to hear someone exclaim twice: 'Shoot him!', evidently meaning me, judging from the menacing talk which followed between the threatener and those with him. I tried to see who the threatener and those with him were, but the street was so crowded I could not. I guessed that they must be gangsters who had mistaken me for another gangster who I coincidentally happened to resemble. I thought one or more of them really intended to shoot me so I hastened from the scene as fast as I could walk.[179]

The onset of voices often seems to be related to specific circumstances and events in the hearer's life. Professor Bleuler himself noted that these experiences 'are usually precipitated by psychic occurrences'.[180] For example, voices sometimes begin after the loss of someone with whom the person had earlier had a significant intimate relationship. Sometimes the voices first appear at a moment of extreme emotional pain, a time when reality may have seemed almost too difficult to bear. In other cases the onset of voices is preceded by a traumatic or emotionally significant event (whether positive or negative) such as an accident, divorce, serious illness or pregnancy.[181]

The Number of Voices

Some people only ever hear a single voice. It may be recognised as someone familiar, although it is frequently not. Often there are two or more voices, in which case a person may hear a dialogue as the two voices discuss him or her. Frequently people hear several voices (possibly of both sexes) which talk or argue among themselves about his or her merits and deficiencies. In such cases, if the voices are all talking at the same time it may be impossible for the hearer to follow everything they are saying. Some people report hearing many voices, as did John Perceval:

> The voices I so often speak of were mostly heard in my head, though I often heard them in the air, or in different parts of the room. Every voice was different, and each beautiful, and generally, speaking or singing in a different tone and measure, and resembling those of relations or friends. There appeared to be many in my head, I should say upwards of fourteen. I divide them, as they styled themselves, or one another, into voices of contrition and voices of joy and honour. Those of contrition were, I think all without exception, on the left temple and forehead; those of joy and honour on the right temple and forehead ... [182]

Frequency of the Voices

Some people only hear voices occasionally or intermittently. Sometimes the voices are only heard when the person is in particular situations or doing certain things. For example, somebody who believes the voices emanate from other people may not hear any voices when there is no one else in their vicinity. Voices are sometimes only heard in conjunction with real, external sounds which the person hears at the same time as the voices. For example, one woman first heard the voice of God talking to her as the clock ticked and later heard voices whenever a tap was running or birds were chirping. Intermittent voices often seem to increase in frequency or intensity during times of stress or emotional arousal. Before the advent of neuroleptic ('anti-psychotic') drugs some people heard voices continuously – perhaps even for decades on end – and some may hardly have had a waking moment free of them. Daniel Schreber has described such an experience:

> For almost seven years – except during sleep – I have never had a single moment in which I did not hear voices. They accompany me to every place and at all times; they continue to sound even when I am in conversation with other people, they persist undeterred even when I concentrate on other things, for instance read a book or a newspaper, play the piano, etc.; only when I am talking aloud to other people or to myself are they of course drowned by the stronger sounds of the spoken word and therefore inaudible to me. But the well-known phrases recommence at once, sometimes in the middle of a sentence, which tells me that the conversation had continued during the interval, that is to say that those nervous stimuli or vibrations responsible for the weaker sounds of the voices continue even while I talk aloud.[183]

Intensity, Clarity and Vividness of the Voices

The voices can range in intensity from being the slightest, barely comprehensible whisper through to the most terrifying, thunderous shout. Their clarity can also cover a very wide range. In some cases the person hears only vague or nebulous sounds, such as a rustling or a confused murmur. However, even if the words of the voices are vague or indistinct, the meaning of what they say is often quite clear to the person hearing them.[184] The voices are sometimes so vivid that they are experienced as sounding just like ordinary human voices. When questioned about the reality of his voices one person said: 'If that is not a real voice then I can just as well say that even you are not now really talking to me.'[185] Another person, when asked if he heard voices, replied:

Yes, sir. I hear voices distinctly, even loudly; they interrupt us at this moment. It is more easy for me to listen to them than to you. I can more easily believe in their significance and actuality and they do not ask questions.[186]

In some instances the voices sound so much like ordinary voices that the hearer simply assumes that they emanate from other people. In the beginning many people presume that others nearby can also hear the voices that they are hearing:

And when I heard voices talking to me, which happened just about every day, I looked around to see if anyone else had heard them too. Sometimes I even asked others if they had heard something, but discreetly enough not to let on what I was hearing. It didn't occur to me that other people didn't hear voices too. Mom had taught me that there were certain things you just didn't talk about. I thought it was the same way with the voices, that all people experienced them in the privacy of their own homes, but like bodily functions, somehow they were a shameful topic not fit for mention in public.[187]

Some people are so utterly convinced of the objective reality of their voices that they do not realise that what they are hearing is purely an inner experience and is not shared by others. The following example illustrates such a case:

The nurse helped me to my room. She asked me if I was hearing voices. She wasn't real. I didn't need to answer her . . . Of course I wasn't hallucinating. The other patients hallucinated but mine was a special case – it may have looked like I was hallucinating but I knew better. Mine was for real . . . All the details were too perfect to have been a hallucination.[188]

Localisation of the Voices

According to a commonly employed clinical rule of thumb voices associated with schizophrenia are typically experienced as coming from *outside* the hearer and are heard with the ears (as ordinary sounds are). Despite its wide acceptance this view is not supported by recent research which has shown that characteristics such as the localisation of the voices and the mode of hearing them are *not* reliably linked to a particular psychiatric diagnosis.[189] In actual fact, where the voices are experienced as coming from and the specific manner by which they are heard vary considerably from one person to another.

Some people living with schizophrenia experience the voices as coming from somewhere in their surrounding environment, perhaps from specific locations such as from behind walls, from within air ducts or ventilators, even from animals, plants, or inanimate objects. Elizabeth Farr suspected that concealed loud-speakers were the source of the voices she heard:

> Many times I would hear them speaking about me as if I were at a cocktail party and I could hear them in the next room. They frequently said things that did not make any sense. For example, I might be walking down the street and hear the words: 'the last stand' coming out of the eaves of buildings. I kept trying to figure it all out. It seemed to me that there must be some unearthly or extra-dimensional power transmitting messages to me through some hidden speakers under the eaves of buildings.[190]

Voices which are localised in the external environment may be heard to come from one side or the other of the hearer, from above or below them, or from behind; interestingly, they rarely seem to come from directly in front.[191] When 'good' and 'bad' voices are localised differently the 'good' voices often seem to come from above whilst 'bad' ones tend to emanate from below.[192] Some people attribute the voices they hear to other people in their vicinity. In such cases the person may deny that he or she is hearing voices and insist, instead, that other people are really talking about them. Sometimes people who hear voices are convinced that others – even if they are very far distant – are also able to hear them. For example, one man who heard long, insulting speeches being made about him believed they could be heard by other people even though they were miles away.[193] In some cases there may seem to be no specific external source of the voices, in which case they may seem to emanate from the sky, or even from some distant part of the universe.

When voices are not localised in the external physical

environment they may be localised within the hearer's own body. Sometimes they are located in one side of the body only. When there are both 'good' and 'bad' voices they may be divided between the two sides of the hearer's body so that the voices are pleasant in the one ear and unpleasant in the other. Many other variations are possible, as Professor Bleuler noted:

> The voices are often localised within the body, mostly for obvious reasons. The mother speaks in the heart or in the ears of the patient; familiar voices are preferably localised in the heart or the chest. Many times, however, the whole body will be intoning, 'You rascal', 'You whore'. A polyp may be the occasion for localising the voices in the nose. An intestinal disturbance brings them into connection with the abdomen; heavy breathing or belching establish a connection with the corresponding organs. In cases of sexual complexes, the penis, the urine in the bladder, or the nose utter obscene words. A really or imaginarily gravid [i.e. pregnant] patient will hear her child speaking inside her womb. One of our patients has a girl in his left hand (with which he masturbates) who speaks to him when he places his hand on his ear. The basis for localisation is not always discoverable. As when a patient hears only his leg talking or when the voices come from various places under the skin, and constantly call out ... Occasionally, the voices are not localised in the body but in the clothing.[194]

While many people are absolutely convinced that the voices they hear are objectively real this is not always the case. Thus, on the basis of such peculiarities as what the voices say, their unusual place of origin, or the invisibility of the speaker, some people are able to differentiate the voices from their ordinary perceptual experiences. People who are aware of the inner subjective origin of the voices sometimes recognise that they are somehow connected to their own thoughts. Some people, unsure if they are hearing actual voices or their own thoughts, have described their experiences as 'voices of conscience', 'audible thoughts', 'soundless voices' or 'thoughts in words'.[195] People who have these kinds of experiences sometimes

describe hearing the voices in their *mind* rather than with their ears.*
As an example, one young woman said of her voices:

> I saw things mocking me from their places, taunting me
> threateningly. And in my head foolish phrases floated
> around without let-up . . . Adding to the torment, strident
> noises, piercing cries began to hammer in my head. Their
> unexpectedness made me jump. Nonetheless, I did not hear
> them as I heard real cries uttered by real people. The noises,
> localised on the right side, drove me to stop up my ears.
> But I readily distinguished them from the noises of reality.
> I heard them without hearing them, and recognised that
> they arose within me.[196]

The specific qualities of voices often change over time. For
example, voices which were initially heard as coming from outside
via the ears may eventually be perceived as located within the
hearer's own head or body.[197] Changes can also occur in keeping
with the hearer's mental and emotional state. Thus, when a person
is stressed or upset their voices may be loud and experienced as
coming from the outside. During times of mental composure, on
the other hand, the voices are often more likely to be experienced
as soft internal whispers which possess only vague auditory qualities. At such times it may be particularly difficult for some people
to say whether they are actually hearing voices or if it is really just
their own 'loud' thoughts.

The Identity of the Voices

It is clear to some people that the voices they hear are a private
perceptual experience which has a subjective origin. Thus, as
explained above, some people recognise that the voices are
somehow connected with their own thought processes: the
'thoughts-out-loud' or 'voices of conscience' and so on are felt to
be internally generated experiences. Some people identify their

---

* Some authorities refer to these kinds of experience as *pseudo*
  hallucinations in order to distinguish them from *true* hallucinations
  which are felt to originate in the external world and are experienced as
  being objectively real (see Slade and Bentall, 1988, p.18).

voices as 'auditory hallucinations' which they accept as being symptoms of schizophrenia (such people are sometimes described as having 'insight' into their 'illness'). On the other hand, some people are so convinced of the objective reality of these experiences that they adamantly refuse to apply such terms to them, as one clinical psychologist discovered whilst working with groups of hospitalised patients who had been hearing voices for many years:

> In no case did patients accept the term hallucinations for these experiences. The term was offensive. It implied they were not real. Almost all patients had private terms of their own for these experiences: The Other Order, The Eavesdroppers, etc . . . There may be one or several figures. Some familiar ones come around day after day, such as one old codger called 'The Old-Timer'.[198]

In some cases visual images may accompany the voices and help to convince the hearer that they must indeed belong to independent beings. For example, one person said that there was a 'voice' perched above each of his ears: 'One voice is a little larger than the other but both are about the size of a walnut, and they consist of nothing else but a large, ugly mouth.'[199] At least at the time of hearing them many people are sure the voices belong to other people, even if they are never actually able to see them. Thus, in one study of a group of people living with schizophrenia, 78% gave a positive response when asked 'Are the emitters of the voices persons in flesh and blood which can eventually be found and seen or touched?'[200] It is not uncommon for people to attribute the voices to others in their environment who they believe are talking to or about them, a conclusion which may sometimes lead to angry accusations being aimed at anyone who happens to be close by when the voices are heard.

The distinctive or peculiar nature and quality of the voices may convince the hearer that something unusual is going on. A very understandable desire to explain their strange experiences may lead some people to develop complex and highly idiosyncratic beliefs about them. For example, some voice hearers may think what they hear emanates from loudspeakers or other types of electronic equipment such as TV or radio. In some cases an unidentified and inexplicable 'influencing machine' operated by unseen enemies with malicious intent is held to be responsible. Some people may even conclude that the source is located within their own body, as was the case with a man who believed the voices emanated from microscopic loudspeakers that had been surreptitiously implanted in his dental fillings.

Voices sometimes seem to have such an intimate knowledge of the hearer's every thought and all the private details of their past history that a supernatural or occult origin is attributed to them. The apparent omniscience and omnipotence of the voices leads some people to conclude that they must be spirits, angels, even God or the devil, or that they have something to do with various psychic or occult influences such as ESP, telepathy or magic.[201] As an example, one man initially attributed the voices of the hostile 'pursuers' he heard around him to real people in his surrounding environment, but when his every attempt to elude them failed he felt compelled to consider other ways of explaining their inescapable and ubiquitous presence: 'The question occurred to me: How could as many of these pursuers follow me as quickly unseen? Were they ghosts? Or was I in the process of developing into a spiritual medium?' Eventually he reached the conclusion that the inescapable voices were produced and broadcast to him by a group of unseen people possessing 'astounding, unheard of, utterly unbelievable occult powers':

> This unique, occult power of projecting their 'radio voices' for such long distances apparently seems to be due to their natural bodily electricity, of which they have a supernormal amount. Maybe the iron contained in their blood corpuscles is magnetised. The vibration of their vocal chords evidently generates wireless waves, and these vocal radio waves are caught by human ears without rectification. Thus, in connection with their mind-reading ability, they are able to carry on a conversation with a person over a mile away and out of sight by ascertaining the person's unspoken thoughts, and then by means of their so-called 'radio voices', answer these thoughts aloud audibly to the person.[202]

The peculiar or even frankly 'bizarre' beliefs which some people develop about the voices may be held with such unshakeable conviction that they reach the intensity of *delusions* (which are also considered to be characteristic symptoms of schizophrenia).

Entertaining such beliefs may eventually lead the hearer further and further from consensual (i.e. shared) reality and ever deeper into a private world known to, and believed in, only by themselves.

People who hear more than one type of voice may identify the various voices differently. For instance, voices which are critical, abusive or threatening may be identified as belonging to evil spirits, negative occult influences, or malevolent unseen enemies, whilst voices which offer praise or encouragement, or which provide guidance or companionship, may be identified as belonging to higher beings or higher parts of the self, spiritual guides, or other mystical or spiritual sources. Interestingly, some people do not contemplate any of these kinds of explanations for their voices but simply hear them without thinking it strange. For example, some people feel that they possess a special ability, such as having 'keen ears' that enable them to hear people speaking all around them, or that they simply have 'the gift of being able to hear things.'[203]

Form and Organisation of the Voices

The speech of the voices may be well organised and quite clear and often consists of short phrases or even single words, although some people hear extensive monologues or engage in long two-way conversations with their voices. Voices quite often take on some special peculiarity. For example, they may speak very slowly or employ rhyming or speak in rhythms. In some cases they may even speak in a foreign language. The voices may adopt various ways of addressing the hearer. Often they talk directly to the person, sometimes even using his or her name. On the other hand, rather than speaking directly to the hearer the voices may speak *about* them. For example, some people hear two or more voices which speak among themselves about him or her (i.e. the voices refer to the hearer in the third person). Many psychiatrists consider these so-called 'third person' voices to be particularly characteristic of schizophrenia.[204]

Some people only ever hear confused or incomprehensible utterances because the voices speak in a disjointed fashion or mention odd phrases which do not seem to make any sense. For example, one person heard a voice state: 'Mary's dog is an ear mother'; another simply heard the words 'sausages and chips' being repeated over and over. Sometimes the voices use unusual expressions which the hearer eventually employs in his or her own speech (such expressions are sometimes referred to as 'neologisms'). It has been noted that the voices of people living with schizophrenia sometimes seem to degenerate over a period of years. In such cases formerly complex sentences may become ever simpler until finally they are reduced to one word or even an inarticulate sound.[205] On the other hand, sentences that were originally quite simple may gradually become more and more complicated and muddled until finally they sound like nothing but 'stupid chattering'.[206] As an example of this, Daniel Schreber has described his own experience of voices which continually repeated the same odd, disjointed phrases:

> The system of not-finishing-a-sentence became more prevalent in the course of the years ... In particular, for years single conjunctions or adverbs have been spoken into my nerves thousands of times ... Thus for years I have heard daily in hundredfold repetition incoherent words spoken into my nerves without any context, such as 'Why not?', 'Why, if', 'Why, because I', 'Be it', 'With respect to him' ... further, an absolutely senseless 'Oh' thrown into my nerves; finally, certain fragments of sentences which were earlier on expressed completely ... [207]

Interestingly, although the voices may have gradually become quieter and emptier over time, sometimes they may regain their original content and clarity during periods of excitement and emotional arousal.

Voice Content

Although what the voices say and talk about can cover a very broad spectrum their utterances often seem to reflect a relatively small number of the hearer's specific hopes, wishes and fears. Certain themes seem to be especially common, most notably those centred on various concerns regarding interpersonal relationships, self-esteem and sexuality. Thus, as Professor Bleuler noted:

> The ambitious hear that power and money are going to be offered them, but certain signs also disclose the manoeuvres of their opponents. The confined patient hears voices that

promise him impending freedom, and others describing his 'imprisonment' as eternal ... The 'voices' of our patients embody all their strivings and fears, and their entire transformed relationship to the external world. The 'voices' are the means by which the megalomaniac realises his wishes, the religiously preoccupied achieves his communication with God and the Angels; the depressed are threatened with every kind of catastrophe; the persecuted cursed night and day ... the 'voices' become, above all, the representatives of the pathological or hostile powers.[208]

The many different names and interpretations which people have given to voices reflect both the very wide range of experiences that are possible and the intensely personal and mysterious qualities these voices often seem to possess. Thus, voices have been called 'communications', 'magical talk', 'secret language', 'rapport', 'voices in uproar', and people have referred to what they hear as 'language magic', 'painful long-distance conversation', 'deadly language', 'cold castigation language' and 'court-of-law punishment language'.[209] The voices of schizophrenia frequently focus on one or more of the following specific themes:

(1) *Threats, Curses and Criticisms*

Threats, curses and criticisms, mostly made in short sentences or abrupt words, often form the main content of the voices. In severe cases critical or accusatory voices may revile everything about the hearer, perhaps criticising them for past misdeeds that never even occurred. Sometimes the voices not only speak but back up their hostile threats by passing electricity through the hearer's body, beating or paralysing him, or taking his thoughts away.[210] Some people feel that the voices know absolutely everything about them and that their faults and shortcomings are being exposed in complete detail by them for everybody to hear. Critical voices sometimes talk about the hearer's innermost thoughts, feelings and memories in such a way as to make them feel that their privacy has been totally invaded. Voices sometimes comment critically on what the person may have just been thinking of doing, possibly even before they are even aware of their own intentions. Elizabeth Farr has described such an experience:

Sometimes I heard the voices speaking my thoughts. They would often think my thoughts before I even thought them ... Many times the voices were harsh with me; they called me obscene names and criticised me unreasonably. Sometimes they yelled and screamed at me and occasionally would wake me up in the middle of the night with such tirades. The voices made it hard for me to concentrate on the things I wanted to do.[211]

Abusive and critical voices often focus specifically on sexual themes. Thus, a woman may hear herself being called a 'slut' or a 'whore', whilst men often find themselves accused of being homosexuals or 'masturbators'. In some instances the voices say such vile things that the person is too embarrassed to reveal the details to anyone. Sometimes voices which have clearly been against the hearer will then contradict themselves and take the opposite position. In such cases the roles of pro and con are often taken by the voices of seemingly different people. In extreme instances a person may be tormented by numerous malicious voices which seem intent on nagging, criticising and completely destroying their self-confidence. One man gave the following description of such an experience:

It is amazing, horrible and for me humiliating, to think what acoustic exercises and experiments – musical ones too – have been conducted with my ears and body for nearly 20 years. Sometimes I could hear one and the same word repeated without interruption for 2 to 3 hours. I had to listen to long continuous speeches about me; frequently the content was insulting and there was often an imitation of well-known persons. These lectures, however, had little truth about them, usually they were infamous lies and slanders about my person, sometimes also of others ... it was often proclaimed that 'I' said all these things ... Sometimes one could only just hear these incessant, uninterrupted sounds but sometimes one could hear them a half or a full mile away. They were being catapulted out of my body and the most varied sounds and noises got slung about ... This is the reason I have been living like a hermit for the last few years. All the time my ears keep ringing and sometimes so loud that it can be heard far and wide. When I am among woods or bushes and the weather is stormy, some horrible, demoniacal poltergeist is aroused; when it is quiet, each tree starts rustling and uttering words and phrases when I approach. So with water – all the elements are being used to torture me.[212]

The identity of hostile or critical voices may be well known to the hearer. However, the quality of the voices sometimes changes or shifts so that the person is left feeling totally confused as to who is really speaking. (As described below, some people hear positive and helpful voices as well as critical and hostile ones. However, during periods of emotional distress, the hostile voices may sometimes become so vociferous that they 'drown out' any others.)

(2) *Running Commentary*

Voices will sometimes simply describe all of the hearer's activities – their thoughts, feelings, or actions – as they occur. For example, a man might hear: 'Now he's combing his hair, now he's getting dressed, now he's walking toward the door', and so on. In such cases the voices will sometimes add critical or mocking comments to their running description, or they might simply *imply* their disapproval by their very tone and manner of expression. Many psychiatrists consider voices which keep up a running commentary to be particularly characteristic of schizophrenia.[213]

(3) *'Thought Echo'*

Some people hear their own thoughts spoken aloud by voices. In such cases the person might hear a voice inside their head simply repeat each thought as they think it or immediately after they have thought it. Sometimes the voice repeating the thoughts is heard to come from the outside and at times it may seem so loud that the person becomes convinced that other people nearby must be able to overhear their every thought so that absolutely no privacy is left to them. Lynne Folkard has described what this can be like:

I believed that the voice could be heard for kilometres around me and that people could listen in. Knowing that my inner and most personal thoughts were being spoken for all to hear was too humiliating to think about and I tried

hard to put it out of my mind ... I reconciled myself to
silence and decided I would never tell another person
anything that had happened to me. If they wanted to know
they could listen in and find out for themselves.[214]

People who have this kind of experience sometimes attribute the
voices to others in their vicinity and become convinced that their
thoughts are being spoken aloud by people around them. Some
people may even hear other people replying to or talking about their
thoughts before they have actually spoken them out loud (which
may lead them to the erroneous conclusion that people are reading
their mind). In extreme cases people sometimes feel that they never
get a chance to think for themselves because they hear the voices
express their thoughts before they have even had a chance to think
them. While they are reading some people may hear the voices read
in advance to them, or if they are about to speak they may hear the
voices get in first and say what they were about to say themselves.

(4) *Commands*

Many people hear voices which order them to do certain things or to
behave in a particular manner. At least initially people who hear such
commands sometimes unquestioningly submit to them, possibly with
unfortunate consequences, as Norma MacDonald has described:

I could eat and sleep very little because of voices telling
me I mustn't. I was 'forced' by voices to walk miles and
miles about the city until my feet were blistered and
bleeding, and then I was persuaded to do an increasing
number of senseless things. [There was] no let-up in the
vicious thoughts that tortured my imagination. Visual and
tactile hallucinations came to enliven the auditory ones.[215]

Although commands issued by the voices often concern behaviours
which are completely harmless (e.g. 'don't use your right hand, use
your left'; 'eat the orange, not the apple'), they may sometimes lead
to self-destructive or suicidal acts and, occasionally, even violence
or aggression. Fortunately, most people are able to resist or ignore
such commands.[216] Nevertheless, some people experience a
protracted inner struggle over whether or not to do as the voices
demand.[217] This struggle can be especially difficult if the voices

attempt to reinforce their authority by threatening dire consequences for refusing to obey. For example, the voices told one woman that she would get cancer if she disobeyed their instructions. In some cases the voices command the person not to reveal their existence or disclose any information about them. If the hearer believes that the voices have a supernatural origin or authority it can be especially difficult to resist their demands, even if they involve out-of-character, dangerous, or even life-threatening behaviour. Elizabeth Farr has explained how she felt compelled to do as the voices commanded, even at the risk of her life:

> I thought the voices came from other worlds. I explained my strange perceptual phenomena as leakage from parallel dimensions. I believed I was approaching an enlightened state. The voices told me that in order to reach this Enlightened state I would have, at the appropriate moment, to jump from the seventh floor of a building and land on my head in a certain way. This would put me at a cosmic junction whereupon my spirit would be taken up from my body and transported to the parallel world where I would receive the ultimate Enlightenment . . . In the light of the fact that my unusual perceptions were extremely real to me and were totally believable, this was not such an off-the-wall conclusion to draw.[218]

Commanding voices are often extremely contradictory. For instance, they may encourage the hearer to do certain things and then criticise them for obeying. Some voices seem to take great pleasure in their ability to confuse or frustrate the hearer and some may even seem intent on driving their unfortunate victim to utter despair with persistent contradictory instructions.* John Perceval experienced this whenever he attempted to eat:

---

* Some people have expressed the opinion that it is actually the voices which cause madness and not the other way around. Thus, the French poet and artist Henri Michaux opined: 'It is not foolishness to say that it is the hallucination which produces madness and not madness which produces the hallucination' (Michaux, 1974, p.60). John Perceval was in little doubt on this matter: 'The contradictory commands were the cause, now, as before, of the incoherency of my behaviour, and these imaginations formed the chief causes of my ultimate total derangement' (Bateson, 1961, p.32).

For at my meals, morning and evening, the voices I used
to hear flocked about me like bees, and every one, in the
tones of some relation or of some friend, begged of me in
turn to refuse a piece of meat for her sake, to leave my
bread for his sake, and so on. Then, when one voice told
me to refuse any thing for her sake, another came to desire
me to eat it for her sake, and I was bewildered.[219]

(5) *Support, Guidance and Companionship*

Although voices are often the cause of great distress many people
also have positive experiences with them. Clinical studies have
shown that some people living with schizophrenia experience their
voices as *predominantly* positive whilst others hear a mixture of
positive ('good') and negative ('bad') voices.[220] For example,
although 58% of one group of people with persistent voices said
that the voices were mainly negative (e.g. abusive, commanding,
accusatory and derogatory), 19% described them as predominantly
positive (e.g. giving instructions or advice, helpful, pleasant,
relaxing, ego-enhancing and anxiety-dispelling). A mixture of both
'good' and 'bad' voices was reported by 29% of the people in this
study.[221]

Intensive studies of the way people feel about their voices
indicate that it is not at all unusual for them to be looked upon as
important personal companions which pay attention to the hearer
and look after them in various ways including protecting and
backing them up, explaining things to them, and teaching them how
to do things. One man explained how his voice felt like a friendly
presence which provided him with comfort, reassurance and
companionship:

It tells me I'm okay if I'm really, really down. Then it's
almost like it's someone there, a friend. So it's okay. That
knows me better than anything else. It's a comfort . . . if it
wasn't there, I'd be like everybody else and lose myself.[222]

Voices can sometimes be helpful and supportive at certain times but
critical or hostile at others. Even when they are predominantly
persecutory they may nevertheless also have certain positive aspects.
Some people feel that their voices have a distinctly beneficial or

therapeutic influence upon them.[223] For example, one woman believed that her voices were created by the Public Health Service to provide her with psychotherapy. In addition to their therapeutic activities the voices advised her on difficult pronunciations and even explained the meaning of various words to her. Other people have described experiencing complex sexual relationships with their voices which result in direct sexual gratification.

Many voice experiences have some kind of religious or spiritual significance to the hearer. For example, during an acute psychotic episode Anton Boisen, the founder of Pastoral Psychology, experienced what he said was 'the most beautiful voice I had ever heard. It was the celebration of the Last Supper.'[224] Professor Bleuler noted that there are times when it can seem as though 'The heavens stand open; the angels and the saints and God Himself communicates with the patient.'[225] The spiritual reality of some voices may be utterly convincing, as John Perceval has explained:

> I heard the voices of invisible agents, and notes so divine, so pure, so holy, that they alone perhaps might recompense me for my sufferings ... I received these as the word of God, for their beauty and their apparent tendency to promote purity and benevolence. And if I doubted, my doubts were overwhelmed if not dissipated by compunction at attributing what was so kind, so lovely, so touching, to any but the divine nature ... [226]

It is quite common for people who hear a number of voices to feel that at least *some* of them are helpful and supportive, even if there are others which are intensely critical or hostile.[227] As an example, one woman divided the voices she heard into the helpful 'Mentors' and the malicious and critical 'Outworlders':

> The two competed for her attention and engaged in heated arguments about what was best for her. When her sewing machine broke and she was unable to fix it, the Mentors gave her detailed step-by-step directions for its successful repair: 'Tighten that screw. Stretch that little spring over there.' They sang songs to her when she was lonely, told jokes, and gave advice as to how to respond to the Outworlders, who would jealously tell her to disregard the Mentors and coax her to commit suicide.[228]

As discussed below, people who experience their voices as being helpful and supportive in some way may be understandably reluctant to comply with treatment regimens (such as neuroleptic medications) which might result in their disappearance. Some people have even expressed the wish for drugs that would selectively eradicate their 'bad' voices but leave the 'good' ones alone!

Responding to the Experience of Voices

There has been an historical tendency to view persons affected by schizophrenia as passive victims of experiences imposed upon them by their condition. In contrast to this prevalent idea in actual fact people living with schizophrenia respond to voices (and to their other experiences) in a highly *active* and *purposeful* way.[229] The style and manner of a particular individual's responses will be influenced by numerous factors including their personal qualities and characteristics, the specific nature of the voice experiences, and their environmental circumstances. Among the factors related to personal qualities of the hearer and their environment might be included:

• The person's individual characteristics including personality traits, emotional maturity, life experience, personal strengths and coping resources;
• The person's age and emotional state at the time the voices began;
• Personal beliefs about the specific identity of the voices (e.g. who the voices are, what their intentions are);
• The person's attitude toward the voices (including what personal meaning and significance they are given);
• The social and cultural context (including the psychiatric milieu) in which the hearer finds him/herself;
• The availability of understanding and appropriate support;
• The concurrent presence of other symptoms (such as non-auditory hallucinations, delusional beliefs, thought disorder);
• The person's level of 'insight' (i.e. the extent to which they can recognise the voices as being a subjective perceptual experience).

Among the factors specifically related to the voice experiences themselves might be included:

• When and how the voices began (e.g. whether onset was gradual

or sudden, whether it was associated with an emotional crisis or came 'out of the blue');
- The specific sensory qualities of the voices such as their intensity, clarity, localisation and vividness;
- The number of voices (e.g. one, several, numerous);
- The frequency and duration of the voices (e.g. whether experiences are brief and intermittent or prolonged and continuous);
- How long voice experiences have been occurring (e.g. a few weeks, several months, many years);
- Specific voice content (e.g. critical, hostile, commanding, friendly, helpful or a mixture of different types of 'good' and 'bad' voices).

Among the very many different ways in which people respond to the experience of hearing voices the following are very common:

Fear and the Urge to Fight or Flee

People who hear voices for the first time during the emotional upheaval of an acute psychotic episode sometimes simply accept them at face value since they assume that others also hear them. Esso Leete had such an experience when she first became psychotic:

> By this time I was hearing voices and responding to them. I was confused, disoriented, and frightened, and remained in a different reality. I made it back to my dorm room, where my room-mate realised something was terribly wrong and comforted me as best she could. Although I was hearing voices for the first time, I truly believed that everyone must hear voices. I thought nothing of it and was absolutely unconcerned. Over the next few weeks I continued to have auditory hallucinations, still not comprehending that I was out of touch with reality as others knew it.[230]

More commonly, hearing voices for the first time is an emotionally moving experience which provokes a powerful personal response. If the voice content is positive the hearer may feel comforted, uplifted or even inspired by it. For example, though she had been deeply depressed, Lynne Folkard was elated by what seemed to her to be a profound spiritual revelation:

As the weeks went by, I did not get any better. I awoke
one morning to hear a voice coming from the back of my
head saying that I would have to serve humanity for the
next ten years. I was very pleased to hear this, believing
that the words in some way represented a spiritual aspect
that had developed in me. I faced each day with a new
sense of well-being. My depression slowly left me and I
gave a great deal of thought to my premonitions.[231]

Especially if it occurs suddenly the onset of voices may be startling
and anxiety-provoking, even if the content is essentially positive.
Many people feel totally perplexed about what is going on and
cannot work out if what they are experiencing is real or if it is 'only
in their mind'. One person described the first moments of her initial
voice experience thus:

On a Sunday morning at 10 o'clock, it suddenly was as if
I received a totally unexpected enormous blow on my head.
I was alone and there was a message – a message at which
even the dogs would turn up their noses. I instantly
panicked and couldn't prevent terrible things from
happening. My first reaction was: What on earth is
happening? The second was: I'm probably just imagining
things. Then I thought: No, you're not imagining it; you
have to take this seriously.[232]

Despite the powerful impact of the initial experience some people
are able to recognise that it involves subjective perceptions which
are not shared by others (i.e. that the voices they hear are an *inner*
experience). In many cases, however, the hearer is initially
convinced that the voices are objectively real perceptions coming
from the outside environment. Depending on the specific nature of
the voices such people may feel fearful about what is happening to
them or angry at those they believe to be responsible. Faced with
an intensely frightening experience some people attempt to flee in
order to escape from those they feel threatened by. One man gave
this description of his own (ultimately futile) attempts to get away
from unseen 'pursuers':

Days later while in the Metropolis again, I was once more
startled by those same pursuers who had threatened me
several days before . . . I heard one of them, a woman, say:

'You can't get away from us; we'll lay for you, and get you after a while!' To add to the mystery, one of these 'pursuers' repeated my thoughts aloud, verbatim. I tried to elude these pursuers as before, but this time I tried to escape them by means of subway trains, darting up and down subway exits and entrances, jumping on and off trains until after midnight. But, at every station where I got off a train, I heard the voices of these pursuers as close as ever.[233]

Sometimes the hearer's initial feelings of panic and powerlessness are followed by a period of great anger toward the voices. Lynne Folkard has described how angry she became when her attempts to free herself from the voice proved ineffective:

The voice in my head reappeared and became so persistent that I wished it would go away. My elation had become resentment. I became aware that I could not control the voice in any way and had lost the power to work out what was sanity and what was not. After several days of this I began to think of ways to rid myself of the voice ... I believed if I spoke to the voice severely he would leave me. I tried a multitude of ways to throw him off ... I sat on my bed calling out for the voice to leave me alone. I suppose I grew more and more vocal. I called out loudly for all to hear that I no longer wished to talk to him, convinced in myself that everyone knew what I was talking about. Eventually, as I became more and more frustrated, I called for him to 'piss off'.[234]

The Search for Explanation and Understanding

If the voices continue and escape proves impossible the hearer faces the challenge of somehow finding a personally acceptable way to make sense of them. The difficulty of this task is added to when voices occur in the context of a psychotic upheaval because at such times there are often so many other strange things going on that it may be extremely difficult for the person involved to think clearly about it all. (In psychiatric parlance it is often said that at such times the person's capacity for accurate 'reality testing' is compromised.) As was explained earlier, people develop various explanations for their voice experiences which make sense to them at the time. Thus, some people may ascribe them to electronic equipment such as TV or radio or else to others in their surroundings who they insist are talking to or about them. Some may conclude that they are being punished for their past misdeeds or present failings and inadequacies. Some people may become convinced that they have been chosen for a special role or mission whose details the voices will eventually make clear. The search to explain strange and unusual experiences may stimulate an interest in occult or supernatural subjects, although this can sometimes lead people to develop unrealistic or even frankly delusional ideas, as Elizabeth Farr discovered:

> In high school I became engrossed in religion, the occult, and the arts as a possible way to help explain what was going on. The central driving feature in my behaviour was to understand my experiences. The delusions started insidiously. I do not know where religion, the occult, and the arts left off and where the crazy ideas started. All I know was that I thought there had to be an explanation for my experiences and I had to be active in my pursuit of an Enlightenment to resolve the conflict between my reality and the reality that everybody else seemed to be experiencing. Everything had to be connected up somehow, I thought. I had to make sense out of it all and connect it up with what I was trying to do in my life.[235]

Experiencing Uncertainty and a Shattering Identity Crisis

People whose voices continue over a long period sometimes remain convinced that their original ideas about them are correct (e.g. that people *are* actually talking about them, or that they *are* being attacked by malicious spirits). On the other hand, many people gradually modify their beliefs as they acquire new ideas or information to apply to their voices. For example, a person might come up with a new theory as a result of reading or seeing a TV programme that describes experiences that seem similar to their own. Although many people are familiar with the fact that there is an association between voices and schizophrenia some people adamantly reject this diagnosis as a possible explanation for their experiences because they are convinced that the voices they hear are objectively real. Lynne Folkard has explained how this can come about:

> The word 'schizophrenia' had never come into my life; I knew nothing of the symptoms and could not believe that the voice in my head was an illness. My thinking patterns seemed normal to me. I stubbornly held to the beliefs and indoctrination the voice was giving me. I suspected that the doctors were not of sufficient intellect to recognise that the voice was real and that they could not recognise his full potential. I went through all the emotions of frustration, shyness, aggression and disgust in the sureness that my voice did exist and could relay through me extremely important messages for humanity ... Deep down in my mind reality did exist for me, and my moments of recognition were of bewilderment at what was happening.[236]

Following an initial period during which they are convinced that the voices are objectively real sounds which emanate from an external source separate from themselves many people gradually begin to question their original beliefs. Even if the voices have stopped the fact that they were heard at all may force the hearer to question the nature of 'reality' and possibly leave them with a deep sense of uncertainty about themself and the world they live in. As he looked back on his own voice experiences (which seemed to involve some type of mind-reading ability), one man asked:

> Do I at the moment believe in telepathy? I can honestly say I do not know, and without there being verifiable scientific proof I will never know. I know quite well that my brain is fully capable of hallucinating any amount of psychic experience for my mind to wonder about; it does so all the time, and this obviously makes it quite impossible for me to assess where my subjective world ends and objective reality begins. I think it is also necessary to ask the question the other way round. How can I be certain that I am hallucinating at all, that what I see when I hallucinate is not a deeper terrible reality of which only a few people are fully aware?[237]

Whatever their original beliefs may have been in time many people do eventually come to understand that the voices are a purely subjective and private perceptual experience. While on one level this realisation may be seen as reflecting the hearer's gradual acquisition of 'insight' it may also herald the beginning of a profound identity crisis. Because hearing voices is widely viewed as an indelible sign of 'madness' throughout Western societies people who have this experience often find themselves struggling with the prospect of having to accept a new view of themselves as someone who is (or has been) 'insane'. Researchers have established that for many persons the experience of voices is an important transitional event which may lead, eventually, to the gradual adoption of a new identity: that of a 'mentally ill' person.[238] One woman has described how afraid she felt as she began to understand the possible implications of accepting that the voices she heard were only in her mind: 'It scared me to death, I thought, well, I'm going completely insane. I'm completely insane. I was more scared than I'd ever been in my whole life.'[239]

The Evolution of Voice Experiences

Over time various developments are possible with respect to voices. Some people only hear them for a relatively short time – lasting anywhere from a few days or weeks to several months – before they eventually stop. Sometimes the voices will disappear spontaneously. Occasionally they might cease quite abruptly, possibly even announcing their imminent departure beforehand, as one man experienced:

> Both my acute episodes were ushered in by the knowledge that I had been communicated with by God ... The whole of my visual field was filled with a brilliant green, I saw the Cross, and then God spoke to me ... The voice continued for four months. One day I was sitting listening to it when it suddenly said the equivalent of 'This is the final transmission: over and out'. I have never heard it since. How did the voice know that it would never come again in spite of a second acute episode?[240]

Rather than a sudden 'switching off' at a specific moment it is much more common for there to be a gradual reduction in the power, intensity and frequency of the voices over time. This sometimes seems to coincide with changes in the hearer's psychological state or in the 'emotional climate' of their living environment, or a combination of the two. Such changes are especially likely to lead to an amelioration of disturbing voices if they result in a generalised reduction in stress and anxiety. A diminution of voice intensity may also be related to the effects of prescribed neuroleptic medications which are presently the cornerstone of the medical treatment of schizophrenia. These drugs may help to diminish the intensity and frequency of disturbing voices, particularly during acute psychotic episodes. However, although it is often claimed that neuroleptic medications are highly effective in eliminating 'positive' psychotic symptoms such as delusions and hallucinations, many people living with schizophrenia continue to hear voices or experience delusional thoughts over extended periods despite their compliance with prescribed medication regimes.* Some highly regarded authorities have estimated that over 50% of people on neuroleptic medications continue to experience 'positive' symptoms to some degree, and that for about 20% of diagnosed persons these drugs have no beneficial effects whatever on these symptoms.[241] (These facts underscore the potential value and importance of effective *non-drug* coping strategies and techniques for people who experience persistent disturbing voices – see Chapter Eight.)

As the voices begin to 'fade into the background' the hearer may find that it becomes increasingly easy to withdraw attention from them or even ignore them entirely. Some people have compared the gradual reduction in the power and influence of their voices to the experience of waking from a dream and subsequently beginning to doubt what was formerly an unquestioned and vivid reality. Regarding this kind of change one woman explained how her voices 'had lost their emotional power and ceased to interest me. The voices said silly things, but were otherwise innocuous.'[242] Another woman told how the influence of her voice had weakened: 'The voice was still there, but it no longer worried me or had the

---

* It is possible that incorrect diagnosis sometimes contributes to this. For example, it has been suggested that some people given a diagnosis of schizophrenia may actually have MPD, a dissociative disorder for which neuroleptic medications are not indicated. These issues are discussed further in Chapter Five.

power over my thoughts it had once had.'[243] A reduction in the power and intensity of the voices sometimes coincides with a movement in the location of their apparent source. Thus, voices which were originally perceived as coming from the outside and heard with the ears may eventually be experienced as located within the hearer's own head or body.[244]

Some people continue to hear voices for extended periods, possibly even for many years. As described below, many people eventually develop effective ways to cope with them or learn to adjust to their continued presence so that they no longer create serious problems. Unfortunately, some people continue to hear voices which cause them great distress. Voices which are persistently critical, controlling or threatening may not only impair the hearer's quality of life and ability to function but also contribute to increasing their risk of substance abuse, self-harm, and even suicide. Researchers have also discovered that some of the so-called 'negative' symptoms of schizophrenia such as loss of motivation and social withdrawal may be a direct consequence of the presence of disturbing voices.[245] For example, in a careful survey in which people were interviewed in their own homes following treatment for acute psychotic episodes, 92% of those who had significant 'negative' symptoms revealed persistent hallucinations or other 'positive' symptoms which were contributing to their on-going need for social withdrawal (e.g. persistent hostile voices made some people too afraid to leave their home). Significantly, many of these people disclosed the presence of their voices only when systematically questioned in their own homes and had been reported as consistently free of 'positive' psychotic symptoms at their aftercare clinics.[246] Even voices which are experienced as friendly or supportive can contribute to social isolation if the hearer becomes excessively involved with them to the extent that he or she begins to lose interest in the outer world of everyday reality. Lynne Folkard has described how she became increasingly absorbed into 'the world of her voice':

The little contact I had with people diminished even further as I moved more and more into the world of my voice . . . I had quite forgotten any attempt to rid myself of the voice and was once again sitting back enjoying what I was being told . . . I contemplated the voice for many hours as I sat on my bed, slowly losing contact with all reality, and putting little importance on what was happening about me. My world had become my relationship with the voice ... I was his 'pretty pretty princess', his chosen one who was to carry out tasks for him. I took my job very seriously, putting vast importance on what he had to say.[247]

Learning to Live with the Voices

People living with schizophrenia who continue to hear voices over a prolonged period invariably go through a process of learning to adjust to their on-going presence. What attitude the hearer eventually takes toward the voices, and what he or she attempts to do about them, will vary greatly from one person to another. For example, while some people engage in a protracted struggle with their voices which may at times resemble a state of intense 'psychological warfare', others learn to simply accept their presence or even establish a personally meaningful relationship with them. The task of learning to live with persistent voices often involves a combination of the following three aspects:

Concealing the Voices

Because hearing voices is commonly seen as a sign of 'madness' many people deny or conceal the fact that they have had such experiences. Even if a person has already received a diagnosis of schizophrenia they may feel disinclined to admit that they are still hearing voices since such a disclosure may result in negative judgements being made about them ('You're still sick'), or lead to unwanted increases in medication dosages or even a return to hospital. (The fact that many people conceal their voices even from the mental health professionals who treat them undoubtedly helps to sustain the questionable perception that neuroleptic medications are highly effective in eliminating hallucinatory voices.) The realisation that others rarely share their convictions about the voices leads many people to conclude that it may be best to simply keep quiet about the whole thing. This is especially likely if the hearer's ideas about the voices are treated with insensitivity or even outright disdain by other people ('They aren't special messages from God, they're just your hallucinations!'). In addition, the voices themselves may instruct the hearer not to disclose their presence, perhaps even threatening dire consequences if they are disobeyed. In some cases the specific content of what the voices say (e.g. scatological or sexual references) may cause the hearer such profound embarrassment that he or she declines to ever speak about it with anyone. Those who have developed a valued relationship with the voices may even be reluctant to breech the confidentiality they feel they have established with them, as Carol North explained:

> I felt creepy talking about the voices. It was like talking behind their backs, except worse because I knew they knew what I was saying about them. I hoped I hadn't gotten them irritated. The consequences could be severe.[248]

Although concealing the presence of voices may help to protect the hearer's self-esteem, it can also have a number of negative consequences, as one person explained:

> Whilst I had to keep the voices a secret I was trapped in my house and my life was dictated by the voices. It used to be scary being so alone, especially when the voices troubled me and had me doubting myself. When I couldn't talk about the voices I didn't know whether what they were saying was true or not . . . [249]

People who experience their voices as positive or helpful in some way may be reluctant to reveal their existence if they believe this will result in them receiving treatment that could weaken the voices or make them disappear.

Learning to Control the Voices

Although they often feel frightened and powerless initially, experience combined with a process of trial-and-error allows most people with persistent voices to gradually acquire a greater sense of control over them. In some cases the hearer's decision to conceal the voices may itself represent their first attempt to regain a sense of control. Early on in their struggle with voices some people may engage in what appear to others to be quite strange or odd behaviours. For example, a person might take the apparently reasonable measure of stuffing their ears in order to block out the voices. Others may invent and enact elaborate rituals or even various kinds of self-styled 'exorcism' in an effort to rid themselves of their invisible tormentors. Unfortunately, some of the techniques that people use in their attempts to control voices may have undesirable consequences. For example, substance abuse or desperate attempts to placate critical or commanding voices by agreeing to do anything they say. Some people have even described trying to deliberately scramble or block their thoughts in order to prevent the voices from listening in on them or speaking them aloud for others to hear (in extreme cases such people may give the appearance of being 'thought disordered').

Many people eventually learn that there are a range of quite simple techniques which they can use to help them cope more effectively with persistent voices. For example, it may sometimes be possible for the hearer to simply ignore the voices or use various distraction techniques in order to put their mind on to something else. The discovery that voices are more likely to occur in certain circumstances than in others allows some people to devise a lifestyle that prevents or minimises their occurrence. Some people find that the most fruitful and effective coping strategy involves selecting the positive or 'good' voices and paying close attention to them while at the same time trying to ignore the negative or 'bad' voices. By using non-drug coping strategies or prescribed neuroleptic medications – or a combination of both – some people eventually manage to eliminate their voices entirely and many others are at least able to minimise the distress and discomfort they cause.

Note: A range of practical strategies and techniques that may help people prevent, alleviate or cope with disturbing voices are described in detail in Chapter Eight.

Developing a Relationship with the Voices

Although the sudden onset of critical or hostile voices is often very frightening and disturbing, over time there are sometimes significant changes in the way these voices are experienced, perhaps even a change in their actual nature. For example, voices which were quite threatening and antagonistic during the emotional turmoil of an acute psychotic episode sometimes seem to become more helpful and friendly later on as things begin to settle down.[250] Mark

Vonnegut has described his own experience of this kind of transformation:

> The voices weren't much fun in the beginning. Part of it was simply my being uncomfortable about hearing voices no matter what they had to say, but the early voices were mostly bearers of bad news. Besides, they didn't seem to like me much and there was no way I could talk back to them. Those were very one-sided conversations. But later the voices could be very pleasant. They'd often be the voice of someone I loved, and even if they weren't, I could talk too, asking questions about this or that and getting reasonable answers. There were very important messages that had to get through somehow. More orthodox channels like phone and mail had broken down.[251]

In time many people seem to evolve a kind of equilibrium with persistent voices so that the early struggle to be rid of them is gradually replaced by a growing acceptance of their presence. In some cases the hearer simply comes to accept – if somewhat reluctantly – that they must learn to put up with and somehow accommodate these 'uninvited guests'. This process may involve a gradual change of attitude toward the voices as the original desire to escape is replaced by curiosity about them and what they have to say. Researchers have found that accepting the voices and trying to learn from them can indeed be an important and effective coping strategy for some people.[252] In fact, people who hear a number of different voices sometimes come to feel that there are at least some which can actually be helpful to them. For example, voices which have been present over a long time may eventually come to be experienced as valued companions with whom a loving and complementary relationship has been established. Nevertheless, the relationships that people living with schizophrenia have with their voices are often characterised by ambivalence and a degree of unpredictable changeableness. Thus, a voice might be valued as an important companion *as well as* being dreaded, or a person might feel sure that even though a voice is sometimes hostile toward them it still likes them.[253] Such voices are often felt to have both 'good' and 'bad' aspects. (In this regard, at least, interactions with them resemble human relations generally since even primarily warm and supportive relationships inevitably involve periods of tension and disagreement!)

The fact that some people develop complex and personally rewarding relationships with long-standing voices leads to the possibility that at times such interactions might tend to become a substitute for ordinary human relations in the everyday world. Many people who have heard voices for a long time *do* become somewhat reluctant to lose them – even if they have mainly been critical or hostile.[254] After all, the on-going presence of voices may have helped to counteract the hearer's feelings of loneliness or isolation or even made them feel special or important ('God cares so much about me that He talks to me personally'). People who have heard voices for many years may have become so familiar with them and so used to having them around that they may become reluctant to give them up even if the voices are sometimes nasty to them. In fact, some people are unwilling to take prescribed neuroleptic medication or use non-drug control strategies because they fear that doing so might weaken or even eliminate their familiar 'old friends'. Anyone who has come to rely primarily on voices for companionship or guidance may eventually begin to depend on them. The challenge of breaking free of such dependency becomes especially important if a person's relationship with voices impairs their ability to function in other areas of life or interferes with their capacity to relate with ordinary people.

Conclusion

The tendency of contemporary mainstream psychiatry to focus almost exclusively on the biological aspects of schizophrenia in both research and everyday clinical practice has resulted in a neglect of the vitally important psychological, social and spiritual aspects of this condition and of the voice experiences associated with it. As a result, with a few notable exceptions[255] the whole question of the personal meaning and significance of the voices of schizophrenia remains virtually unexplored. In this climate the negative aspects of voices have tended to be over-emphasised and treatment regimens usually limited to attempts to alleviate the diagnosed person's problems by eradicating their voices. However, as the first-hand descriptions in this chapter have shown, for many people living with schizophrenia hearing voices is a complex and multi-faceted experience which has both negative *and* positive aspects. That the presence of hallucinatory voices does not necessarily result only in undesirable consequences for the hearer is suggested by research which compared various characteristics of people living with schizophrenia according to whether or not they experienced hallucinations. Interestingly, not only were those who experienced hallucinations found to be no more socially isolated than those who did not, they were also judged by their peers to be more friendly and likeable, less defensive and more wanted as room-mates.[256]

Voices do undoubtedly cause great distress to many people living with schizophrenia, both because of their specific contents and as an indirect consequence of the fact that hearing them may itself be a source of fear and embarrassment. Difficulties associated with troublesome voices have probably been exacerbated by the long-standing tendency in psychiatry to view people who have a diagnosis of schizophrenia as relatively passive 'victims' who are capable of doing little to help themselves apart from 'complying' with prescribed neuroleptic medication regimes. This attitude has resulted in very little interest being shown in understanding and fostering the capacity of diagnosed persons to do things to help themselves with voices and other problems. Fortunately there are signs that this historical trend is at last beginning to change, as is reflected in recent attempts by some researchers to formally investigate the many ways in which people living with schizophrenia strive actively to cope with and overcome their difficulties.[257] As more is learnt about these frequently unrecognised and untapped potentials it is likely to become increasingly clear that in the future a major role of mental health professionals and other helpers will be to provide encouragement and support to diagnosed persons as they discover effective ways of helping and healing themselves.

Paying closer attention to the voice experiences associated with schizophrenia throws open a window onto a number of possibilities which warrant serious consideration. At the very least it raises questions which are often consigned to the proverbial 'too hard' basket. For example, why is it so common for people with this diagnosis to attribute their voices to 'spirits' or some other kind of supernatural entities? Why are the voices so often extremely hostile (some seem to be downright malevolent), and why do they frequently seem fixated on sexual and scatological matters? How is it that some voices appear to possess knowledge or wisdom far exceeding that of the hearer? And how is it possible to account for those occasional voices which seem to demonstrate an uncanny ability to predict future events? This list could be extended indefinitely. The chapters that follow are devoted to a consideration of a number of issues which will hopefully begin to furnish answers to some of these difficult but important questions.

Chapter Five

MULTIPLE PERSONALITY DISORDER

*Such a doubling or multiplication of the self can take place
that patients find themselves confronted by entirely alien
forces, which behave as if they had a personality . . . The
fact that such phenomena are possible remains of the utmost
importance for any evaluation we may make of the human
psyche and its nature.*

– Karl Jaspers[258]

Among the various mental disorders in which voices can occur as
a significant feature, Multiple Personality Disorder is undoubtedly
both the most extraordinary and the most challenging. There is also
growing opinion that it may be far more common than has
previously been realised. Although a great deal still remains to be
learnt much progress has been made in recent years by researchers
striving to lay the foundations for a scientific approach to further
investigation of this complex and difficult area. This important work
began with the development of unambiguous definitions and clear
guidelines for diagnosing this mysterious syndrome.

The American Psychiatric Association has defined Multiple
Personality Disorder (MPD)* as a dissociative disorder characterised by the presence within a person of two or more distinct
identities or personality states which recurrently take control of the
person's behaviour. The number of separate 'personalities' (often
referred to as 'alters') which can coexist in someone with MPD
ranges from two to more than one hundred, although about half of
all reported cases involve ten or fewer.[259]

Psychiatrists have long known of this disorder but until quite

---

* In 1994 the American Psychiatric Association adopted the term
  'Dissociative Identity Disorder' to refer to what was formerly called
  Multiple Personality Disorder (see APA, 1994).

recently most considered it to be extremely rare. Outside the world of psychiatry popular fictional accounts of individuals who supposedly had more than one personality (such as in Robert Louis Stevenson's famous story of *Dr Jekyll and Mr Hyde*) have contributed to making the notion of a 'split personality' familiar to most people.* In 1957 the first real-life case of MPD to capture public and professional attention was described in *The Three Faces of Eve*, a book in which two doctors related their account of the diagnosis and treatment of a woman with three distinct personalities.[260] Popular awareness of this phenomenon was greatly increased with the publication in 1973 of *Sybil*, a best-selling book later made into a popular Hollywood film which told the story of a woman who had sixteen alter personalities.[261] In 1993 Joan Casey described her extraordinary life with over two dozen alter personalities in *The Flock*, the first autobiographical account of MPD.[262]

The American Psychiatric Association listed Multiple Personality Disorder in its diagnostic handbook for the first time in 1980 thereby officially recognising it as a mental disorder. Since then there has been a dramatic increase in the number of people given this diagnosis with an estimated 20,000 new cases being reported between 1980 and 1990.[263] At the same time there has been a veritable explosion of professional interest in MPD and other dissociative states as reflected in the formation of an international association (The International Society for the Study of Multiple Personality and Dissociation), the publication of a number of specialist journals (e.g. *Dissociation*), and the establishment of regular conferences, seminars and training workshops for therapists, researchers and other interested parties. Research is still in its infancy and there are a great many differences of opinion regarding the validity of MPD as a discrete mental disorder. Nevertheless, one psychiatrist who is a widely recognised authority believes that 1% of the general population in urban North America might be affected by this syndrome and that between 2% and 5% of all psychiatric

---

* Interestingly, Robert Louis Stevenson claimed that many of the details of this novel were dictated to him by the 'little people' of his dreams. The tendency of both dream characters and fictional literary creations to act as though they were autonomous beings with ideas and feelings of their own is discussed in Chapter Six.

in-patients and a 'substantial number' of out-patients may have full-blown undiagnosed MPD.[264] Women appear far more likely to develop MPD than men and they also tend to have a larger number of alter personalities with an average of fifteen or more compared to about eight for men.[265]

MPD as a Survival Strategy

It is now widely accepted that in the vast majority of cases people diagnosed with MPD have survived severe and prolonged traumatisation in childhood.* Identified sources of trauma include extreme cultural, religious or political persecution, war, famine and natural disasters. In most of the cases so far diagnosed in North America prolonged physical and/or sexual abuse (often incestuous) has been identified as the primary contributing factor. As one authority has put it: 'What is MPD? MPD is a little girl imagining that the abuse is happening to someone else.'[266]

To the extent that it is helpful to the victim MPD can be looked upon as a creative strategy for coping and surviving in exceptionally difficult circumstances. For a child (most often a girl between the ages of 4 and 6) faced with extremely unpleasant or even emotionally and physically intolerable experiences, the creation of a fantasised companion may be a source of desperately needed comfort and relief. The following scenario illustrates how this might sometimes begin with the abuse victim imagining the voice of a reassuring friend:

> Her voice first appeared at age ten when she was lying in bed at night, alone and terrified after another incestuous attack . . . She said she felt so incredibly alone that it was unbearable, and she made up a 'friend' who began to comfort her. Her conversations with this 'friend' grew more

* This may not necessarily be true of *all* cases of Multiple Personality Disorder, however. Although severe childhood trauma is very common among those who come into therapy it is possible that both the symptoms and causes of MPD may be different in non-clinical populations. Ryan and Ross (1988) found that MPD can also occur in persons with no history of childhood physical or sexual abuse.

frequent and more complicated as time and the abuse went on.[267]

Many authorities believe that when the distress of prolonged abuse is severe, continuous and inescapable some victims are able to unconsciously create entire personalities (alters) whose characteristics and functions depend on the person's particular needs at the time. For example, alter personalities may embody powerful emotions which are too painful for the young abuse victim to tolerate (e.g. anger, rage, fear, pain), or they may have strengths or skills the abused person wishes to possess:

One example is a personality who explained, 'I came to help when she was raped. She needed someone to take over. I don't like sex but I can manage it, I'm a whore and a prostitute but she [the victim] is very moral and proper. I'm a tramp, just dirt and filth, but I can take over the sexual part of life which she can't tolerate'.[268]

The fact that a person with MPD is not simply pretending or faking is supported by clinical observation and scientific research which has established that the various alter personalities can have vastly different characteristics, many of which would be extremely difficult if not impossible for anyone to consciously control or manipulate. For example, alters can differ in terms of their brain wave profiles (as measured by EEG), sensitivity to drugs (e.g. differential response of blood glucose to insulin), medical status (e.g. symptoms of asthma, sensitivity to allergens), visual acuity (colour blindness, need for eyeglasses), pain tolerance, and left or right-handedness.[269] There have even been cases reported in which no withdrawal symptoms were evident when an alter heavily addicted to heroin switched to a non-addicted personality.[270]

Researchers have found that for a long time (often many years) most people with MPD are unaware of the existence of their 'other' personalities due to the presence of a complex state of amnesia that effectively forms a barrier between them. Thus, even though a person may have begun developing alter personalities early in childhood, MPD is usually not suspected or diagnosed until the affected person is well into adulthood. Furthermore, while many people imagine that MPD involves a sudden and dramatic switching between one alter personality and another such as might be portrayed in a scene from a 'Jekyll and Hyde' type movie, this does *not* necessarily occur although it can. Observers – professionals as well as family members and friends – may therefore fail to appreciate the true underlying explanation for the person's erratic behaviours:

> Cases of multiple personalities vary from blatant examples where personalities are frequently on display, to subtle cases where personalities can only be identified with certainty via hypnosis. Nevertheless, some of these 'subtle' cases have later revealed as many as 50 personalities. Transformations . . . are frequently occurring in these patients but the casual observer will see, for example, only tearful, angry, or childish behaviours. Hypnosis will then reveal personalities as the responsible agents . . . Personalities may take over the body at times but they are usually latent.[271]

Often all the affected person and others are aware of is a range of odd or unusual feelings and experiences which cannot readily be explained. Most people with MPD experience a number of the following:[272]

• Inability to remember childhood or recall important personal information (which cannot be accounted for by ordinary forgetfulness);
• Frequent blank spells (often lasting from seconds or minutes to hours or days, though some people have had amnesic episodes for years at a time);
• Headaches (often followed by a blank spell);
• Suddenly 'waking up' and finding themselves in an unfamiliar place or with strangers after a blank spell;
• Feelings of unreality (depersonalisation);
• Flashbacks (reliving past events as if they were presently happening);
• Noticing that things (including money) are missing or discovering objects in their possession (such as items of clothing) but having no idea where they came from and how they got there;
• Hearing voices (usually coming from inside the head).

Because the diagnostic significance of these non-specific symptoms is often underestimated (they are frequently likely to be attributed to another disorder such as schizophrenia), many authorities feel that systematic inquiry about them should always be a routine part of psychiatric assessment. Special questionnaires and structured interview schedules have been developed for the specific purpose of reliably determining the presence of dissociative disorders including MPD.[273]

MPD and Voices

Sometimes the only awareness a person with MPD has of the various alter personalities that coexist within them is the experience of hearing the voice(s) of one or more of the alters speaking in their head. As an example, for a long time before she was eventually diagnosed as having multiple personalities Christine Sizemore (whose experiences formed the basis of the famous *Three Faces of Eve* case mentioned above) had been hearing a voice she couldn't explain. It was this voice that was her primary concern and her original reason for seeking professional help:

> On one of Chris's visits to the doctor, she abruptly left the subject they were discussing and asked, 'Doctor, does hearing voices mean you're going insane?' She looked at him intently. 'What do you mean, "hearing voices"?' he asked. 'Hearing them in your head when there's nobody there.' Her eyes dropped. 'Well, why don't you tell me about it? Have you been hearing voices?' ... 'Yes. And they come from inside my head.' 'How do you know they come from inside your head? Perhaps they are coming from behind you?' 'No, they're not. There's nobody there. And anyway, it doesn't sound like it's behind me. I can tell it's inside my head.' 'Perhaps you're just thinking out loud. Maybe you just spoke your thoughts aloud,' he suggested. 'No. My voice comes out here, at the front.' She touched her lips. '*This* voice speaks inside my head. And anyway, I wouldn't ever think what it says.'[274]

The initial phase of MPD therapy involves a therapist making contact with the various alter personalities and then helping the diagnosed person to gradually begin the process of recognising and starting to reintegrate these dissociated aspects of him/herself. Before this can be done, however, there is often a complex 'amnesia barrier' in place which prevents a person with MPD from being aware of the existence of the alters. In most cases all he or she may be aware of apart from the unexplained blank spells, headaches and other non-specific symptoms is that they hear voices. Hearing such 'inner' voices is a very common experience for people with MPD. In a recent study of a group of 236 persons with this diagnosis 71.7% reported hearing voices arguing and 66.1% heard voices commenting.[275] A very wide range of variation exists in the nature and quality of the voices. Sometimes they are commanding and persecutory and may even order the person to harm themself or others. They may specifically forbid the hearer from revealing information about them or the alter personalities. In some cases the voices may be soothing and reassuring. Sometimes the voices discuss the hearer while referring to him or her in the third person (i.e. as 'he' or 'she'). Voices are sometimes reported to converse with one another, to scream, cry, and squabble like babies or small children.[276] MPD therapists often use hypnosis in order to make initial contact with the alters that are responsible for the voices, as in the following example:

> One patient heard voices intermittently for years telling her, 'You are no good,' or shouting, 'You never stand up for yourself.' They later proved to be those of two personalities, Carol and Esther. Another patient kept hearing a female voice that cried, 'You're stupid!' Under hypnosis, I spoke to Mabel (a personality), who blithely admitted that she was the culprit.[277]

The Identity of the Alters

The various secondary or alter personalities that exist in a person with MPD are seemingly created from memories, feelings, wishes and drives which have become dissociated or 'split off' from the original or 'core' personality. In some cases there may be only a few such alters (Eve had two), while in others there may be many (Sybil had sixteen). Since MPD originates in the many different aspects of a *single* person alter personalities are not actually separate people, although the complex psychological processes which are involved may result in the creation of a range of quite diverse, seemingly separate individual personalities, including some which may be of the opposite sex to that of the core personality. There are usually a number of alters which act to protect or help the core personality. Among the different types of 'protector' personalities there may be some that are quite active while others provide help by what they know rather than by what they do. For example, some may simply observe whatever is happening and maintain an awareness of all the other alters. Many therapists feel that helper personalities – which are sometimes referred to as 'Inner Self-Helpers' or ISHs – can play an important role in the process of healing and reintegration:

> The 'inner self-helper' ... is a rational, usually all-knowing, mature personality that serves as a guide for the therapist and the patient. The 'inner self-helper' often acts as an ally of the therapist ... suggesting new avenues of treatment, or giving the therapist clues to hidden memories or personalities whose conscious realisation would be therapeutic for the patient as a whole. The inner self-helper is sometimes a wise old man or teacher that claims it is chronologically older than the actual age of the patient.[278]

In addition to the 'protectors' many people also have 'persecutor' alters which carry out hostile attacks on the other personalities using both physical and psychological means. Persecutors often seem to be the instigators of suicide attempts, 'accidents', self-destructive and self-defeating patterns of behaviour and various kinds of out-wardly directed aggression. Although they may appear to be extremely hostile or even malevolent (in one research study 28.6% of the persecutor personalities actually claimed to be demons[279]), some MPD therapists believe that their underlying motivation is often positive (e.g. euthanasia is a common rationale for them urging the host to suicide). Some persecutors may actually be helpers using self-destructive strategies:

> They often present as tough, uncaring, and scornful, but this is usually just a front for an unhappy, lonely, rejected self-identity. One persecutor I worked with was abusing the other personalities because she felt rejected, because she felt they did not appreciate the hard work she did holding

all the anger, and because they were always blaming her for everything that went wrong.[280]

In some cases an alter personality may be identified as that of a dead relative or even of someone who is still alive. In such cases the alter may be experienced either as a protector or a persecutor according to the type of relationship the core personality had with the person in question (for example, a formerly nurturing grandmother may be identified as a protecting alter). Some research has shown that many people with MPD also have alters which they identify as 'discarnate entities' of various kinds including dead people from long ago, spirit guides, astral entities, psychic intrusions or undifferentiated beings of uncertain origin.[281]

MPD and Schizophrenia

Although it may have originated as a desperate coping and survival strategy, MPD is nevertheless a disorder which can create many problems in the affected person's life and in the lives of others, including family and friends.* It is hardly surprising, therefore, that most people with MPD have a lengthy history of involvement with mental health services. However, as a consequence of the fact that it is only relatively recently that MPD has begun to be recognised and accepted as a legitimate mental disorder, many people with multiple personalities are likely to have received a range of *other* psychiatric diagnoses from the professionals they have had contact with. Researchers have established that most people are likely to have been involved with the mental health system for seven or eight years before MPD is finally diagnosed, and that most will have received an average of three or four different psychiatric diagnoses during that time, the most common being a mood disorder, borderline personality disorder, and schizophrenia.[282]

A number authorities believe that MPD is commonly misdiagnosed as schizophrenia. For example, one researcher found that 40.8% of a group of 336 persons finally diagnosed with MPD

---

* On the other hand, it is possible that some individuals with MPD maintain an ability to function at a high level and show no evidence of pathology in their everyday lives (see Kluft, 1986).

had previously been given a diagnosis of schizophrenia.[283] The reason this occurs may be related to the fact that there are many similarities between the symptoms that most psychiatrists consider to be characteristic of schizophrenia and those associated with MPD. As was pointed out in Chapter Four, voices which keep up a running commentary or two or more voices which converse with each other are usually considered to be key diagnostic criteria for schizophrenia. However, some researchers believe that voices commenting and voices arguing are also two of the most common MPD symptoms. Furthermore, many of the so-called 'Schneiderian First-Rank Symptoms' which psychiatrists often consider to be diagnostic hallmarks of schizophrenia actually appear to be even more common in people with MPD.[284] Thus, in a group of 47 persons diagnosed with MPD, in addition to hearing voices (47%), many reported feeling that their mind was being influenced (38%) or controlled (36%), that they were being plotted against (31%) or followed (27%), or that their thoughts were being broadcast (22%) or stolen (20%).[285] It has been suggested that the widespread acceptance of schizophrenia as a diagnosis has contributed to the lack of recognition of the legitimate status of MPD during the course of this century.[286]

In order to differentiate between MPD and schizophrenia skilled professional assessment by a person familiar with *both* disorders is necessary. The following factors have been suggested as clues which raise the possibility that MPD may be an appropriate diagnosis:[287]

- A history of childhood sexual and/or physical abuse;
- A history of non-specific MPD symptoms such as blank spells, headache, and feelings of unreality (see the list above);
- Self-destructive behaviour (e.g. multiple suicidal gestures or attempts, persistent self-injury);
- Previous diagnosis of schizophrenia or borderline personality disorder (or both);
- Failure to respond adequately to conventional treatment for schizophrenia (i.e. neuroleptic medications) despite adequate trials;
- Absence of thought disorder;
- Absence of so-called 'negative' symptoms of schizophrenia (e.g.

loss of motivation, blunting or flattening of emotions, poverty of thought);
• Hearing voices inside the head (see below).

Talking with the Voices

Anyone acquainted with the 'good' and 'bad' voices so commonly heard by persons living with schizophrenia is likely to find descriptions of protector and persecutor alters (including reports of demons, spirits, and various other 'discarnate entities') strangely familiar. As a general rule, it seems that people with multiple personalities hear the voices *inside* their head. Some authorities have suggested that another distinguishing characteristic is that it is often possible to talk with MPD voices. Indeed, one psychiatrist who is an authority on multiple personalities believes that mental health clinicians should always attempt to make contact with and speak to their patient's voices *whatever* psychiatric diagnosis has been given:

> In the routine clinical assessment of auditory hallucinations one should determine whether it is possible to talk to the voices ... It is important for the examiner to think about the voices *as if* they were actual people and try to find out what they are like, what they are doing, and what their motivation seems to be. In other words, one should examine *all* auditory hallucinations as if they come from alter personalities, in order to positively rule dissociation in or out. This applies no matter what the clinical diagnosis.[288]

In implementing this approach the therapist is advised to begin by asking the person to simply describe the voices (e.g. the number of different voices, their sex, whether they are friendly or hostile, what they say, the tone and manner of their speech, and so on). Following this the therapist may attempt to interact with the voices themselves:

> It is often possible to engage MPD voices in an indirect conversation. To do this one explains to the patient that one wants to try to talk to the voice. One then asks the voice a question, the voice answers, and the patient reports what the voice said. It may be necessary to identify the voice being addressed in the following way: 'I want to ask the

voice that Mary says sounds like a little girl a couple of questions. I want the voice to answer, and Mary will tell me what the voice said. First I want to know if the voice that sounds like a little girl can hear me.' If the patient answers that the voice said, 'Yes,' one then proceeds with further questions.[289]

Some psychiatrists used this type of approach in an investigation of the voices of a group of 45 psychiatric patients with a range of different diagnoses (31 had a diagnosis of schizophrenia) in order to learn what percentage may have had multiple personalities. Using hypnosis they were able to contact and engage in conversation with the 'voices' of many of these patients. They concluded that 60% had previously unidentified 'alter' personalities which were responsible for their voices. Of the 31 persons who had a previous diagnosis of schizophrenia, 20 were identified as having multiple personalities.[290]

While these exploratory approaches can be very informative attempting to distinguish between the voices of schizophrenia and those of MPD on the basis of whether or not it is possible to speak with them is not necessarily a simple or clear-cut matter. Thus, for example, it may not be possible to speak with the voices in so-called 'polyfragmented MPD' since the numerous alters in such cases appear to consist mainly of multitudes of personality 'fragments' rather than discretely functioning personalities. On the other hand, some therapists have described holding rational conversations with the voices of people who have been reliably diagnosed with schizophrenia, as the following example illustrates:

I examined a young native [American Indian] man with schizophrenia. He had numerous severe negative symptoms, inappropriate affect, poverty of speech and movement, a psychotic sister, and a supportive, warm, non-abusive family. But I could talk to his voices. He had two main voices with whom he held conversations. Both spoke in English and were white, although other minor voices spoke in Cree. He described one as good and one as bad. The bad one wanted him to assault people and generally act in an unpleasant manner. The good one tried to soothe him and advised more socially acceptable behaviour. The bad one sometimes claimed to be the Devil . . . I had a long rational conversation with the two voices. They both gave their points of view on the patient and each other, spoke politely, and would be described as 'cooperative to examination' in a classical mental status examination report. The voices in this patient were more than chaotic symptoms of insanity. They were in fact sane.[291]

Cases such as this highlight the possibility that some people may have both MPD *and* schizophrenia or a borderline personality disorder, a possibility which many MPD therapists accept.[292] On the other hand, it may indicate that the voices of schizophrenia are sometimes the result of a process of 'splitting off' of mental contents in a similar fashion to that which occurs on a massive scale in MPD. (This theory and others regarding the possible origins of hallucinatory voices are discussed in detail in Chapter Six.)

The Outcome of MPD Therapy

Despite the fact that MPD can be a seriously disruptive and disabling disorder most authorities agree that it can be *cured* with skilled psychotherapy provided by experienced MPD therapists (a claim which is supported by the outcomes of the various cases documented in the first-person accounts mentioned in this chapter). Indeed, one leading authority has stated that there is no other psychiatric disorder of comparable severity which has such a good prognosis.[293] Nevertheless, there is some disagreement among therapists as to what the most desirable outcome of therapy actually is. On the one hand, some therapists aim to achieve 'fusion' and the development of a unified sense of self-identity by eliminating the separate selves altogether. On the other hand, there are therapists who feel that a more creative outcome for the person with MPD is the attainment of a state of 'integration' involving harmonious cooperation and communication between the various alters which remain active as a network of close and valued friends.[294] A rather similar question may arise with respect to persistent voices generally, whatever context they may happen to occur in. One of the important issues which will be addressed in Chapter Nine concerns the question of whether an attempt should be made to eliminate voices entirely or whether it might not sometimes be better for a person to learn to accept and live in harmony with them.

Conclusion

Although it has been formally recognised as a legitimate mental disorder for nearly two decades MPD continues to generate much controversy. Many mental health professionals remain sceptical about it and some have even suggested that certain therapists may be unwittingly *creating* multiple personalities in their highly vulnerable clients by subtle forms of suggestion and reinforcement. Concern has also been expressed about the possibility that some people may be capable of having vivid recollections of traumatic events that never actually occurred (this has been termed the 'false memory syndrome'). Scepticism about MPD is undoubtedly partly based on the fact that for a long time the huge numbers of people given this diagnosis in North America had not been found in other parts of the world, which led to the suggestion that it might even be a culture-specific syndrome. However, serious doubt was cast on this assertion with the publication in the *American Journal of Psychiatry* in 1993 of the results of the first large scale study to be done outside of North America. This research established that persons diagnosed with MPD have a stable set of core symptoms which are strikingly similar whether they reside in North America, the Netherlands or elsewhere in the world.[295]

Some mental health professionals simply deny the existence of MPD altogether while others continue to insist that it is at best very uncommon. Thus, as recently as 1988 one popular book on schizophrenia described MPD as 'an extremely rare condition' declaring furthermore that 'none of the symptoms of schizophrenia are normally found in such patients'.[296] As the research cited in this chapter has shown, the claim that symptoms usually attributed to schizophrenia are not found in persons with MPD is not supported by available clinical evidence. Indeed, not only does this assertion fly in the face of research it also contradicts the views of two of the most eminent authorities on schizophrenia in the world. Thus, Professor Eugen Bleuler, the Swiss psychiatrist who coined the term schizophrenia, was of the opinion that 'schizophrenia produces different personalities existing side by side'.[297] Professor Manfred Bleuler, also a distinguished international authority, has expressed

a very similar view: 'This impressive phenomenon of two personalities in one patient, of the split personality, is one of the
justifications for the label schizophrenia'.[298] It is safe to say that
over the past two decades evidence has been accumulating which
appears to be at odds with the long-standing notion that dissociative
disorders and schizophrenia are completely distinct and unrelated
clinical entities.

Professional resistance to considering the possibility that MPD
may be a valid dissociative disorder is likely to be partially related
to the fact that widespread acceptance of the existence of such a
trauma-induced syndrome would pose a serious challenge to the
hegemony of the biomedical model which attempts to explain
mental disorders in terms of putative biological malfunctioning of
the brain.[299] There is also an understandable though morally
inexcusable reluctance to acknowledge the terrible reality of
childhood physical and sexual abuse, the high frequency of which
among adult psychiatric patients is still largely unrecognised and
inadequately investigated.[300] On a more general level, many people
feel distinctly uncomfortable in considering the possibility that
under certain circumstances a sufficiently distressed human being
may be capable of 'fragmenting' into numerous autonomously
functioning personalities. At the same time, however, many people
experience a curious fascination with the phenomenon of MPD –
as the huge popularity of books and films such as *The Three Faces
of Eve* and *Sybil* indicates. Could it be that in these very extreme
cases we see a dramatically intensified reflection of the 'multitude
of selves' that secretly exist within every human being? Research
into the nature of consciousness would appear to confirm such an
intuition. Dr Roger Walsh, one of the world's leading authorities
on this subject, has pointed out just such a possibility:

> Multiple personalities provide a dramatic example of
> dissociation and divided consciousness. However, the
> implications of research on dissociation are much more
> subtle and extensive. They suggest that all of us live with
> some degree of dissociation and that 'the unity of
> consciousness is illusory'. The implication is that anyone –
> ancient shamans, modern channellers, and all the rest of
> us – may be capable of receiving information from aspects
> of our own psyches that lie outside conscious awareness.

This information may seem to come not from our mind but from another entity, a fact that can be easily demonstrated with hypnosis. Some of the communication may consist of information and memories that the conscious personality has long forgotten. When this occurs the effect can be particularly dramatic and provide apparently impressive evidence that the message must come from another entity.[301]

Belated recognition of the importance of dissociation has opened up many new avenues for exploring the various ways in which early traumatisation can contribute to the subsequent development of psychopathology. Furthermore, while there continues to be uncertainty regarding its status as a valid mental disorder, there is little doubt that the extraordinary phenomenon of MPD raises many challenging and important questions about the nature of consciousness and the human psyche's seemingly ever-present capacity for adaptation and transformation. More specifically, it highlights the extent to which a degree of dissociation and 'multiplicity' may be the norm for every human being.

Note: Readers wishing to find out more about MPD and other dissociative disorders are advised to consult the Recommended Reading section at the end of this book and/or to contact one of the growing number of groups providing information, support and referral (see Appendix).

Chapter Six

THE ORIGIN OF VOICES

We can understand the true nature of inner voices only if we
recognise that these are a heterogeneous group of
experiences. A continuum of inner voices exists which
includes both hallucinations and revelations.

– Mitchell Liester[302]

Any attempt to account for how and why people hear voices is bound to be fraught with difficulty. The most obvious reason for this is the fact that the experience of hearing voices covers such a wide range of diverse possibilities that no single explanation could ever hope to fit all situations. Indeed, even the most intricate theorising would probably still be unable to account for the many individual variations and nuances that are possible. A few moments reflection on the contents of the previous chapters makes it abundantly clear that voice experiences cover an impressively broad spectrum, ranging from the quite common and rather innocuous 'normal' experience of hearing one's name called when alone, through to the sublime and inspiring experiences described by many saints and mystics which may also constitute a cherished aspect of the spiritual lives of some more ordinary folk. Even the voice experiences which have undoubtedly received the greatest attention from psychologists and researchers – those associated with schizophrenia – involve a dauntingly complex array of different possibilities which range from incessant, hostile attacks through to those providing the hearer with an invaluable source of comfort, reassurance and companionship.

This chapter aims to provide an introduction to a wide range of different views regarding the origin of voices.* It must be

---

* In most cases the theories outlined have been somewhat simplified for the sake of clarity. Readers who are interested in a more detailed and comprehensive account are urged to consult the original references and the resources listed under Recommended Reading at the end of this book.

emphasised that the theories outlined below are offered as ideas to think about rather than as definitive answers or complete explanations. Furthermore, there may well be other hypotheses about voices which are just as valid in specific cases as the ones listed here. Some voices may be best accounted for by more than one of these hypothetical mechanisms or by various combinations of them. It should also be understood that there might be considerable overlap between some of these hypotheses and that more than one might apply in any particular case. It is possible, for example, that in addition to hallucinatory voices people with a diagnosis of schizophrenia might also have other voice experiences which are unrelated to their psychotic condition (e.g. 'bereavement' voices). Finally, it is probable that some of these theories may be more specifically applicable to voice experiences which occur in the context of mental disorder while others may apply to voices which occur in non-psychiatric contexts.

Before proceeding with a discussion of specific theories it is important to emphasise that hallucinations exist on a continuum with 'normality' and that any and every intermediate gradation of experience is possible. At the 'normal' end of this hypothetical continuum are ordinary thoughts and ideas ('I thought'). Next are thoughts which are experienced as having a degree of autonomy, as if they came from somewhere else ('It occurred to me'). Further along are the vivid imaginings and inspired thoughts which are clearly felt to have a quality of 'otherness' and which are often personified ('A little bird told me'). Included here are the familiar 'voice of conscience' and various other 'inner voice' experiences. Such experiences gradually shade off into those which have a vaguely sensory quality ('It was *as if* someone spoke to me'). Then there are experiences which are convincingly sensory but still heard internally ('I hear a voice speaking in my heart'). Finally, there are some voices which are experienced as being clearly sensory and fully externalised ('I hear a voice outside me speaking quite distinctly').

A good part of the difficulty that inevitably arises when discussing voices relates to the fact that many people have experiences which do not fit neatly into a particular category (e.g. 'I'm not sure if it's a voice or my own thoughts'). Some psychiatrists recognise that this uncertainty is quite common among people who have a specific psychiatric diagnosis such as schizophrenia.[303] Thus, many people may say that what they experience is like a thought but that it becomes so intense at times that it then seems to be more like a voice. The possibility that some voice experiences may change in a fluid and dynamic way in accordance with the hearer's state of mind and circumstances should be kept in mind when considering the theories listed below.

1 *Self-Talk*

Everyone speaks to themselves in their own mind. This so-called 'self-talk' often involves statements a person makes to him/herself about what they are experiencing, feeling, doing or planning to do, and so on. A lot of self-talk is emotionally neutral. For example, a person might simply talk to themselves about what they are seeing (e.g. 'The sky is becoming very grey. I wonder if it's going to rain?'). A person's self-talk is often coloured by the frame of mind they are in. Thus, the self-talk of someone who is feeling happy will frequently involve positive self-statements (e.g. 'My new haircut makes me look really good'). Critical self-talk, on the other hand, involves a person saying things to themselves which have a rather negative or pessimistic tone. Up to a point this kind of self-talk can serve the useful purpose of helping to prevent mistakes or other undesirable behaviour (e.g. 'Better slow down! If I keep driving this fast I might get booked for speeding'). Unfortunately, critical self-talk sometimes becomes *intense* and *obsessive*, in which case a person may end up spending a lot of time berating and putting themselves down (e.g. 'I'm really stupid', 'No one really likes me', 'I've never been good at anything', 'I'm a total failure'). For some people critical self-talk may have begun at a very early age. For example, a young child experiencing constant intense criticism from significant others may eventually 'take it on board' and begin saying to themselves the kinds of things they originally heard other people saying to or about them.

Some voices may begin as self-talk. For example, while most people easily recognise that the so-called 'voice of conscience' is actually their own conscience 'speaking' to them, a person experiencing intense guilt feelings (such as often occurs during a period of severe depression) may forget its inner origin and consequently feel as if they are being tormented or accused by a voice which comes from somewhere outside of themselves. Self-talk can become so intense and persistent at times that it may seem to take on a life of its own thus leaving a person vulnerable to attack by personified self-doubt or self-criticism. Hostile and attacking voices which have evolved out of a person's intensely negative and critical self-talk can be very destructive because of the way they continually work to undermine the hearer's self-esteem and self-confidence. People who hear such voices sometimes seem to forget how they began and become convinced that it is really *other* people who are saying terrible things about them.[304] By contrast, voices which have developed from positive self-talk may be comforting and reassuring – much like the 'imaginary companions' that many young children have.

Although there may be times when they are quite convinced that others *are* speaking about them (during an acute psychotic episode, for example), many people living with schizophrenia eventually come to recognise the inner origin of their voices. They may subsequently refer to them as 'loud thoughts', 'thoughts in words', or use other terms which reflect the fact that they are recognised to originate in their own thought processes.

2 Subvocal Speech

Some people unconsciously whisper to themselves while they are reading or concentrating intensely on what they are thinking about. The hypothesis that voices may sometimes originate in self-talk is supported by research in which it has been found that *some* people living with schizophrenia whisper softly to themselves while they are hearing voices and that what they are whispering subvocally sometimes corresponds closely with what they hear the voices saying.[305] In such cases the hearer and the speaker (i.e. the voice) are actually one and the same person! Loneliness and lack of social contact might contribute to this behaviour. Thus, as one person said of his own experience of hearing voices:

> I am quite positive it is caused by a lack of conversation – opportunities to speak to people. If a person doesn't have the opportunity to speak to someone he will speak to himself. To speak is a natural desire; when that desire is suppressed it must come out some way or another.[306]

The fact that some people are able to stop their voices by using simple physical strategies that occupy their vocal chords, lips and tongue (as described in Chapter Eight) adds support to the notion that some voice experiences may originate in subvocal speech.

3 *Imagination*

People who hear voices are sometimes told (often rather dismissively) that they are just 'imagining things'. Although it is certainly impossible to account for *all* voice experiences in this way it is quite likely that some voices do actually originate in the imagination of the hearer. Psychologists have long recognised that certain people have such an extremely vivid imagination that they are able to conjure up images (i.e. pictures, sounds, smells, sensations) which are so life-like they are experienced as if they were actual sensory perceptions of the physical world. The ability to create such images (which is called *eidetic imagery*) is quite common in children and, although it often disappears during adolescence, may be retained by some adults, as the writer George Bernard Shaw affirmed:

> There are people in the world whose imagination is so vivid that when they have an idea it comes to them as an audible voice, sometimes uttered by a visible figure.[307]

For many creative individuals the ability to imagine vividly is a very important source of inspiration. One of the most intriguing things about the creations of the human imagination is that at times they may seem to have a life – and possibly even a mind – of their own, a characteristic which many writers are familiar with. Some authors have even described having to make substantial alterations to plots or storylines because they discovered that their fictional characters didn't seem to want things to develop in the way the writer had originally planned! Playwrights, poets, and novelists often claim that the characters in their developing works 'speak because they want to speak', sometimes surprising them with what they have to say. As an example, Alice Walker has described how writing her novel, *The Colour Purple*, entailed a year of speaking with and listening to the various characters as they told her their story:

Just as summer was ending, one or more of my characters – Celie, Shug, Albert, Sofia, or Harpo – would come for a visit. We would sit wherever I was, and talk. They were very obliging, engaging, and jolly. They were, of course, at the end of their story but were telling it to me from the beginning. Things that made me sad often made them laugh. Oh, we got through that; don't pull such a long face, they'd say.[308]

Although most people do not have an imagination quite as vivid as this, everyone has some capacity to create characters with their own mind. Such imaginal characters can range from those which have no distinctive qualities (appearance, feelings, beliefs, etc.) apart from those which have been consciously given to them, through to those which speak, feel and act in ways that seem to be completely autonomous and independent of the person imagining them. Characters resulting from the activity of *autonomous imagination* often have the mysterious quality of seeming to originate from outside of the imaginer:

A special kind of imaginative capacity operates outside conscious awareness. It is in touch with levels of mind and body outside the reach of conscious control. At the same time, it is in touch with the external, cultural environment, and responsive to it. This distinctive mode of imaginative construction is capable of drawing on information not present in the individual's consciousness – information derived from both internal and external sources – and shaping it into an imaginative product (dream, vision, automatism), which then emerges into the individual's consciousness in the form of imagery as seemingly external to the self as the images of sensory perception. The reality of its products, we should note, is neither that of the external, cultural world nor the inner world of one's conscious thoughts and feelings, but something else again, something that weaves the two into a third world, a world as imagined. Yet it is not a realm of consciously contrived imagining, but one that is independent of the conscious self.[309]

Some voices may originate in the imagination of the hearer as a form of wish-fulfilment (although the person concerned may be creating them quite unconsciously), as in the following example of a woman who had been hearing the voice of her mother:

> 'The voices make me feel bad, but I also enjoy them in a way. I seem to look for them like an old, lost friend.' She compared her looking for the voice to looking for her late grandfather to reappear. 'I look around, sort of expecting him to come out of the room again as he did when alive.' 'I knew by the way the voices answered it couldn't just be my conscience. ... The voices too were constantly telling me what to do just as if a mother were talking to a child. *I guess I wanted a mother so badly I just imagined one.*'[310]

Carl Jung believed it was possible to learn from the various figures of the imagination, whether they are consciously created in deliberate fantasy activity or spontaneously produced in dreams. He developed the technique of 'active imagination' as a way of engaging, talking with and learning from such imaginal figures. (Jung's own profoundly enriching experiences in dialogue with an imaginal character he named 'Philemon' are described below.)

4 *Dreams*

Hallucination-like experiences are a key feature of dreams. Indeed, Jung declared that 'dreams are the hallucinations of normal life.'[311] All human beings routinely see and hear things in their dreams that are not actually present in the outer world of physical reality. In other words, a dreamer has sensory experiences which lack an appropriate external physical stimulus – which is precisely how hallucinations are defined. Furthermore, while a person is dreaming they don't just *think* they are seeing or hearing things – they actually *do* see and hear them in a way that is just as vivid and real as are ordinary waking sensory perceptions. Only when a person awakens do they realise they were 'only' dreaming and that what they experienced does not correspond to external reality.

The mechanism of *projection* gives dreams one of their most intriguing characteristics: the quality of seeming to come from outside of the dreamer. Projection is a psychological process by means of which a person unconsciously attributes his or her *own* characteristics (e.g. attitudes, feelings, thoughts, etc.) to other people. (Projections can also be made onto animals or inanimate objects – such as ink-blots, as in the famous Rorschach test, which psychologists use to analyse a person's projections.) Thus, when a person hears a voice speaking in a dream it seems to belong to someone else, to a person separate and distinct from the dreamer themself. This occurs despite the fact that what is being said and heard actually originates from within the dreamer's own mind. Dreams are sometimes likened to plays since they often involve a 'cast' of characters each with his or her own 'speaking part':

> The actors appear, the roles are distributed; of these, the dreamer takes only one that he connects with his own personality. All the other actors are to him as foreign as strangers, although they and all their actions are the creation of the dreamer's own fantasy. One hears people speaking in foreign languages, admires the talent of a great orator, is astounded by the profound wisdom of a teacher who explains to us things of which we do not remember ever having heard.[312]

Since voice experiences are often felt to be objectively real and frequently also have this peculiar quality of 'otherness' they have been compared to dreams. It has been suggested, for example, that some voice experiences are like fragments of dreams which have somehow intruded into the hearer's waking consciousness. In such cases the voice-hearer may be likened to a person who is 'dreaming whilst awake'.

5 Internalised Memory-Images ('Introjects')

Everybody carries in their mind memory-images of persons who are or were significant to them. Put simply, people we have known (or aspects of them) live within us in our memory and, to a greater or lesser degree, can be recalled at will simply by thinking about the person concerned. For various reasons these memory-images are sometimes partially or even completely hidden from conscious awareness (for example, by being deeply buried in the unconscious part of the mind), in which case they cannot readily be accessed, although they may reappear spontaneously from time to time in dreams or other altered states of consciousness (e.g. hypnosis, active imagination).

These internalised images (which are sometimes called 'introjects') may be relatively true to life and thus constitute an accurate record of what the person concerned is (or was) actually like and how they really did behave. On the other hand, such inner images may be based more on the way a person was perceived to be rather than how they actually were, in which case their memory may be rather exaggerated or distorted. For example, a young child's tendency to experience the world in 'black and white' terms often means that others are perceived to be *all* good or *all* bad. Consequently, a person may carry an idealised image of a parent or other figure which is so perfect that it is actually 'too good to be true'. Some internalised memory-images may be based more on qualities or characteristics a child *wished* parents had possessed than on their actual characteristics. In some cases internalised memory-images involve highly negative exaggeration or distortion so that the person in question is recalled as being terrible – perhaps even evil – in a way that is really quite unrealistic. Sometimes the image of a single person may become split into two opposite parts (e.g. a 'good' and a 'bad' mother). It is also possible for the identities of several different persons to become fused together as a result of a psychological process called 'condensation'.

Some voices may be related to internalised memory-images. In such cases the voices are likely to be experienced as belonging to a *person* (in contrast to those which are heard as simple disembodied statements which are more akin to 'loud thoughts'). According to the theory of Transactional Analysis (TA), everyone has at least four or five 'people' in their head. For example, we may have 'internalised' a number of people who had a significant influence on us when we were growing up. In addition to our parents, we may have internalised other influential relatives, school teachers, close friends, and various role models. Proponents of TA believe that adult behaviour is often strongly influenced by the wishes or commands of such internalised people and is communicated via their remembered voices. Dialogues with 'inner people' are believed to occur on a number of different levels or degrees:

> In the first degree the words run through [a person's] head in a shadowy way, with no muscular movements, or at least none perceptible to the naked eye or ear. In the second degree, he can feel his vocal muscles moving a little so that

he whispers to himself inside his mouth ... In the third
degree he says the words out loud ... There is also a fourth
degree, where one or other of the internal voices is heard
as coming from outside the skull. This is usually the voice
of the parent (actually the voice of his father or mother)
and these are hallucinations.[313]

Voices which develop on the basis of introjects can have a number
of possible functions. Sometimes they may be significant sources
of comfort, reassurance and guidance to the hearer. For example,
experiences in which a deceased person is felt, seen or spoken with
may originate as a way for the bereaved person to maintain a sense
of contact with a departed loved one. Internalised memory-images
may even be experienced as faithful inner companions, as one
woman explained:

I feel like there's a person inside me, a male, and we talk
to each other. Sometimes it goes on all day, we just talk as
if he was walking beside me. He's so real, and I can even
hear his voice, a male voice. I'm very lonely, and I would
miss him if I didn't talk to him. Now I talk to him about
once a week, maybe twice a week. It used to be every day,
24 hours a day and I'd get so tired.[314]

Some disturbing voice experiences seem to involve *intrusive* and
involuntary recollections of aspects of negative internalised memory-
images.[315] In some ways this is similar to the way past memories
(whether they are pleasant or unpleasant) can spontaneously re-appear
in dreams, except that the voices are heard while the person remains
fully awake.

6 *Personified Projections ('Autonomous Complexes')*

The fact that disturbing voices frequently involve themes such as
criticism, anger and sexuality suggests that they may originate with
thoughts, feelings or wishes which, for one reason or another, are
unacceptable – perhaps even intolerable – to the person who has
them. As an example, a person with very low self-esteem may have
reached a point in their life when they are tormented by deep
feelings of inadequacy, failure and self-reproach. Such a person's
'self-talk' may have become extremely negative and critical. If it

reaches an intolerable emotional intensity an automatic and unconscious process of *dissociation* may occur which provides a degree of respite. Dissociation is a psychological mechanism by means of which certain aspects of the psyche are 'split off' from conscious awareness and ego-control and begin to function independently. Thus, for example, a thought such as 'I hate myself' may become dissociated and projected into the outer world. By this means the unbearable feelings are externalised.

As a result of the operation of the mechanisms of dissociation and projection a person who was once tormented by self-accusation may come to feel themselves accused by *others*, possibly in the form of threatening and accusatory voices.* Such a transformation of inner conflicts into voices provides some relief for, as painful as it is to be accused or reviled by others, it is not as unpleasant as it is to accuse and be unacceptable to *oneself*. In fact, when such a transformation occurs a person who previously felt intense self-hatred may experience an increase in self-esteem. They may feel, for example, that they are being *falsely* accused by the voices and that they are actually completely innocent of everything they are accused of.[316]

As well as specific thoughts or feelings it is possible that entire *psychological complexes* formerly present in the unconscious mind may be 'split off' (dissociated) and projected outwards. In Jungian psychology a complex is defined as a constellation of psychic elements such as ideas and opinions which have become grouped together around a specific emotionally charged theme. The so-called 'inferiority' complex is a well-known example. Dissociated and externally projected aspects of the self such as complexes are invariably *personified* through a psychological process similar to that which occurs regularly in dreams. Thus, projected thoughts, feelings, or wishes may reappear in the form of one or more *persons* suffused with the 'disowned' qualities (e.g. if an individual habitually refuses to acknowledge their angry feelings they might have a dream in which they are confronted by a violent person intent on destruction). As well as being personified 'split off' complexes

---

* It is interesting to note, in this regard, what Professor Eugen Bleuler said about the persecutory voices so often heard by persons with a diagnosis of schizophrenia: 'In many instances the persecutor is nothing else than the personification of the patient's conscience.' (Bleuler, 1950, p.405)

frequently attain a high degree of autonomy.* While the presence of autonomous complexes is often most evident in states of mental disturbance, Jung insisted that far from being an abnormal phenomenon the psyche's tendency to dissociate was an inherent aspect of its nature:

> Let us now turn to the question of the psyche's tendency to split. Although this peculiarity is most clearly observable in psychopathology, fundamentally it is a normal phenomenon ... The tendency to split means that parts of the psyche detach themselves from consciousness to such an extent that they not only appear foreign but lead an autonomous life of their own. It need not be a question of hysterical multiple personality, or schizophrenic alterations of personality, but merely of so-called 'complexes' that come entirely within the scope of the normal.[317]

Jung believed that the distinctive qualities of the voices of schizophrenia were due to the presence of dissociated and personified autonomous complexes:

> Activated portions of the unconscious assume the character of *personalities* when they are perceived by the conscious mind. For this reason, the voices heard by [people living with schizophrenia] seem to belong to definite personalities who can often be identified, and personal intentions attributed to them. And in fact, if the observer is able ... to collect together a fair number of these verbal hallucinations, he will discover in them something very like motives and intentions of a personal character.[318]

Anxiety-provoking ideas or feelings are not the only raw materials from which personified projections are created. Jung believed that images from the unconscious which are encountered in dreams often help to compensate for conscious attitudes which are rigid or maladaptive and that voices may sometimes serve a similar function. Jung noted, for example, that people living with schizophrenia

---

* The fact that some voices can actually be 'interviewed' (see Chapters Five and Seven) is an indication of the extent of their highly developed autonomy and 'personhood'. Jung referred to personified autonomous complexes as 'fragmentary personalities' or 'splinter psyches'.

occasionally hear voices which correct them or chastise them for indulging their unrealistic delusional ideas. (This notion is discussed further in Chapter Nine.)

Although it has historically been seen as a pathological (abnormal) phenomenon a growing body of evidence supports the view that partial or mild degrees of dissociation may be quite normal.[319] Sleepwalking is an example of a normal dissociative state in which the ordinarily unconscious part of the mind temporarily takes control of a sleeping person's behaviour while the conscious aspect of their mind remains unaware of what is happening. Many children probably utilise a mild degree of dissociation in order to create the 'people' who become their imaginary companions. In certain circumstances dissociation may serve important adaptive purposes. For example, in situations of extreme isolation some people may unconsciously call upon their capacity to dissociate to create 'hallucinatory' companions to keep them company (some examples of this were discussed in Chapter One). While dissociation is seen in its clearest and most extreme form in Multiple Personality Disorder (which, as was discussed in Chapter Five, may itself be an adaptive strategy), a lesser degree of a similar phenomenon also occurs in normal dreams, fantasy activity, creative imagination and altered states of consciousness.

7 Sub-personalities

Whether it is manifested in dreams, fantasy, creative activity or hallucinations the capacity to create 'new' personalities is at least partially dependent on the fact that the human personality *already* consists of many separate, semi-independent 'sub-personalities' which fit together like a complex jigsaw puzzle to form the unique individual that every person is. Rather than consisting of aspects of significant others which have been taken in (such 'Internalised Memory Images' were described above), these sub-personalities may be an inherent aspect of every human being's psychological make-up. Thus, for example, during an inner conversation it is possible for a person to become aware of the fact that different parts of themselves seem to hold different views and may even take different sides in an argument. Careful self-observation leads to the realisation that the various 'parts' actually have their own personality and view of life. Thus, each sub-personality has a style, an attitude and a set of beliefs of its own and can function almost as if it were a 'person' in its own right. For instance, the so-called 'inner child' may represent the innocent part of a person (or in some cases the frightened, angry or hurt part that is carried deep inside). Some common sayings reflect the fact that a person can be under the influence of one or more of their sub-personalities even though they may only be vaguely aware of their existence. For example, a person may say they are 'in two minds' about something when two sub-personalities are vying for control. On the other hand, someone may say they don't know 'what got into them' when a particular sub-personality has temporarily taken control without their awareness. The fact that various sub-personalities can have very different – possibly even quite contradictory – attitudes and traits is a potential source of conflict unless a person is able to develop an awareness of their presence and an understanding of the extent to which they exert an influence on behaviour:

> Each of us is a crowd. There can be the rebel and the intellectual, the seducer and the housewife, the saboteur and the aesthete, the organiser and the bon vivant – each with its own mythology, and all more or less comfortably crowded into one single person. Often they are far from being at peace with one another. As Assagioli [founder of Psychosynthesis] wrote, 'We are not unified; we often feel that we are, because we do not have many bodies and many limbs, and because one hand doesn't usually hit the other. But, metaphorically, that is exactly what does happen with us. Several sub-personalities are continually scuffling: impulses, desires, principles, aspirations are engaged in an unceasing struggle.'[320]

Most people are only ever vaguely aware of the range of sub-personalities that exist within them. However, under highly stressful circumstances (such as may occur during the distress of an acute psychosis, for example) the 'voices' of sub-personalities may be experienced quite vividly. In such instances a person may even have a lively conversation, argument or debate with a sub-personality without ever realising that they are actually talking with an unrecognised part of themselves. Some voice experiences may even involve a person 'listening in' as a conversation or discussion takes place between two or more of their sub-personalities.

A number of methods have been developed to help people become more aware of the presence and influence of their sub-personalities. Specific approaches include Psychosynthesis[321], Transactional Analysis[322] and Voice Dialogue.[323] The two Jungian therapists who devised the Voice Dialogue approach maintain that in a very real sense 'multiple personalities' are a natural part of every human being's psychology and that techniques such as theirs simply help to bring them more clearly into awareness:

> Voice Dialogue introduces awareness into our psychological make-up . . . From this still point, the drama played out by the subpersonalities and the ego is clearly visible . . . Subpersonalities, or voices, are constantly operating within everyone. As we have stated earlier, they are the energy systems that experience life. Voice Dialogue gives us a chance to objectify them, name them, understand them, and work with them creatively. When we use Voice Dialogue, we are sensitising ourselves and others to the drama played out by these subpersonalities.[324]

A person's various sub-personalities may be helpful or harmful or both. For many people the sub-personality with the greatest destructive potential is one which is sometimes referred to as the 'inner critic'. In the following clinical vignette a Voice Dialogue facilitator addresses the voice of the 'inner critic' of a woman named Janet, thereby clearly illustrating the extent of its hatred and hostility:

> *Facilitator:* I was wondering about how you feel toward Janet. You criticise her all the time about her looks and her lack of accomplishment, and every time you say something, she freezes up and can't get anything done.
> *Critic* (with real venom): I don't care. She's better off dead than living in that half-assed fashion. I despise her and, frankly, I don't care if I kill her. She deserves to die, the creep![325]

Most people are subjected to occasional attacks by an 'inner critic' sub-personality, though fortunately these attacks are usually relatively mild. However, in its more extreme form this kind of hostile and destructive inner voice is highly reminiscent of the critical voices often heard by persons with a diagnosis of schizophrenia.

8 Archetypes of the Collective Unconscious

As a result of his pioneering psychological research Carl Jung formed the opinion that, as well as consisting of a *personal* unconscious of hidden (repressed) memories and wishes, the human mind (or psyche) also has a much deeper level which he termed the *collective* unconscious. Jung felt that just as the physical body has a very long evolutionary history so too does the mind, the collective unconscious being that part of it which retains and transmits the common psychological inheritance of humankind as a whole. Jung referred to this level of the unconscious as 'collective' because he felt that within it were to be found the deepest roots from which all human experience ultimately arises:

> The collective unconscious is better conceived as an extension of the personal unconscious to its wider and broader base, encompassing contents which are held in common by the family, by the social group, by tribe and nation, by race, and eventually by all of humanity. Each succeeding level of the unconscious may be thought of as going deeper and becoming more collective in its nature. The wonder of the collective is that it is all there, all the legend and history of the human race, with its unexorcised demons and its gentle saints, its mysteries and its wisdom, all within each one of us – a microcosm within the macrocosm.[326]

Jung found that the collective unconscious contains a wealth of primordial images which he termed *archetypes*. Archetypal images can manifest themselves in a variety of ways and when they do they are invariably personified (the tendency of psychic contents to assume the guise of 'persons' was described earlier). Personified archetypal images give rise to the basic forms taken by the various gods and goddesses of religion, the heroes and heroines of mythology, the innocent or evil characters in fairytales, and the extraordinary and beguiling figures encountered in dreams. The Wise Old Man, the Great Mother, the Miraculous Child, the Hero/ Saviour, and the Trickster are just a few of the many archetypes of the collective unconscious. Jung especially emphasised the psychological significance of the archetypes he called Anima (the image of the feminine carried within a man's psyche), and Animus (the masculine image carried within a woman's psyche).*

Jung observed that when archetypal images become manifest they always exert a very powerful effect upon consciousness. The conscious mind, which usually experiences them as if they came from the *outside*, may fall under their influence as if under a magical spell:

> [T]he archetypes have, when they appear, a distinctly numinous character which can only be described as 'spiritual', if 'magical' is too strong a word . . . In its effects it is anything but unambiguous. It can be healing or destructive, but never indifferent . . . This aspect deserves the epithet 'spiritual' above all else. It not infrequently happens that the archetype appears in the form of a *spirit* in dreams or fantasy-products, or even comports itself like a ghost. There is a mystical aura about its numinosity, and it has a corresponding effect upon the emotions. It mobilises philosophical and religious convictions in the very people who deemed themselves to be miles above any such fit of weakness. Often it drives with unexampled passion and remorseless logic towards its goal and draws the subject under its spell, from which despite the most desperate resistance he is unable, and finally no longer even willing, to break free, because the experience brings with it a depth and fullness of meaning that was unthinkable before . . . The essential content of all mythologies and all religions and all 'isms' is archetypal.[327]

Archetypal images are sometimes encountered in dreams. Dreams which contain this kind of imagery have a powerful, deeply moving and unforgettable emotional impact on the dreamer. Such experiences, which are rooted in the collective unconscious, are sometimes referred to as 'big' dreams in order to distinguish them from more

---

* In Chapter Nine the hallucinatory experiences of a man named Joe are described. Teresa, the young woman whose voice Joe heard and whose image he saw, may have represented an externalised personification of Joe's *anima*.

ordinary dreams which originate primarily from the level of the personal unconscious. States of acute psychosis also often involve a wealth of archetypal imagery. Thus, in a relatively common scenario a psychotic individual may experience him or herself as being at the centre of a 'cosmic' battle between powerful universal forces of Good and Evil or Light and Dark, while at the same time being impelled on some heroic journey or mission upon whose outcome the fate of the entire world depends.[328]

Many of Jung's most penetrating insights into the nature of the psyche came about as a result of his fearless exploration of his own psychological depths. During his investigations into the nature of the unconscious Jung experienced in fantasy a vivid encounter with the Wise Old Man archetype in the form of a 'guiding spirit' he named Philemon. The two engaged in animated conversation and Jung, accepting that Philemon knew things of which he himself was profoundly ignorant, tried to remain open and receptive to instruction. Jung's experience with 'Philemon' and other archetypal figures was especially noteworthy for the fact that they seemed to exist outside of him and have their own independent and autonomous reality. As a result of such experiences he concluded that the psyche was not merely a subjective phenomenon but that it consisted also of an *objective* aspect (this he called the 'objective psyche'). In his autobiographical memoir Jung said of his imaginal encounters:

> Philemon and other figures of my fantasies brought home to me the crucial insight that there are things in the psyche which I do not produce, but which produce themselves and have their own life. Philemon represented a force which was not myself. In my fantasies I held conversations with him, and he said things which I had not consciously thought. For I observed clearly that it was he who spoke, not I. He said I treated thoughts as if I generated them myself, but in his view thoughts were like animals in the forest, or people in a room, or birds in the air, and added, 'If you should see people in a room, you would not think that you had made those people, or that you were responsible for them.' It was he who taught me psychic objectivity, the reality of the psyche. Through him the distinction was clarified between myself and the object of

my thought. He confronted me in an objective manner, and I understood that there is something in me which can say things that I do not know and do not intend, things which may even be directed against me. Psychologically, Philemon represented superior insight. He was a mysterious figure to me. At times he seemed to me quite real, as if he were a living personality. I went walking up and down the garden with him, and to me he was what the Indians call a guru.[329]

At the end of his long and extraordinarily productive life Jung steadfastly maintained that all of his most important psychological insights had their origin in the profoundly moving fantasies and dreams which he explored during the early part of his career. It was his firm conviction that in the autonomous creations of fantasy, imagination and dreams, in religious experiences, in psychotic states, and in ordinary wakefulness, the wisdom of the unconscious often speaks to the conscious self in the form of voices and visions.

9   *Paranormal Phenomena*

During the past one hundred years many cases have been reported of voice experiences which appear to involve premonitions, extrasensory perception (ESP), telepathy and various other kinds of so-called 'psychic phenomena'. The practices of mediumship and trance channelling (described in Chapter Two) involve the deliberate use of supposed psychic abilities to obtain information that would otherwise be inaccessible. In addition to these kinds of activities some people have reported *spontaneous* experiences which appear to involve paranormal perception. Although many 'psychic phenomena' involve a person knowing something *directly* without the mediation of voices or any other kind of sensory impression, researchers have nevertheless collected numerous examples of experiences in which voices have played a key role. These, together with a great deal of other evidence, lend strong support to the reality of paranormal phenomena.

Despite the fact that many people seem to have had at least one mysterious and apparently paranormal experience at some time during their life a great deal of controversy still surrounds this subject. It is interesting to learn, therefore, that there has been serious scientific interest in the whole field of what has come to be called 'parapsychology' since at least the latter half of the nineteenth century. The Society for Psychical Research, established in England in 1882, was the first body formally dedicated to the study of psychic phenomena. A distinguished Cambridge University philosopher, Professor Henry Sidgwick, was one of its founding members and William James, a philosopher and psychologist from Harvard University, helped to organise an American Society for Psychical Research, established in Boston in 1885. James, who is often considered to be the founder of modern psychology, served as president of the Society and in 1909 published a collection of writings entitled *Essays in Psychical Research*.[330] In modern times rigorous academic research continues to show that many people believe they have had some kind of paranormal experience. For example, among the 300 staff and students who responded to a survey conducted in 1987 by Dr Peter Nelson of Queensland University's Department of Studies in Religion, 82% said they have had such experiences.[331]

In the 'Census of Hallucinations' conducted by Professor Sidgwick and his colleagues for the Society for Psychical Research (see Chapter One), some respondents described having had experiences in which information was conveyed to them by a voice in seeming contradiction of the laws of ordinary physical reality. As an example, the following anecdote involving a premonition mediated by a voice was reported by a vicar who, following a meeting at an inn with a group of sailors, had agreed to join them early the following morning to sail in their boat to a nearby island. The vicar prepared for bed fully intending to go with the sailors, but his plans were unexpectedly interrupted as he was on his way upstairs to his room:

> I had got up about four or five stairs when someone or something said, 'Don't go with those men.' There was certainly no one on the stairs, and I stood still and said, 'Why not?' The voice, which seemed as if some other person spoke audibly inside my chest (not to the ear), said in a low tone, but with commanding emphasis, 'You are *not* to go.' 'But,' I said, 'I have promised to go.' The answer came again, or rather I should say the warning, 'You are *not* to go.' 'How can I help it?' I expostulated,

'they will call me up.' Then most distinctly and emphatically the same internal voice, which was no part of my own consciousness said, 'You must bolt your door.' All this time I stood still on the staircase ... On reaching the room I lit the candle, and felt very queer, as if some supernatural presence was very near me ... At the very last moment (it was quite a toss-up which it should be) I bolted the door and got into bed. A great calm succeeded the past agitation, and I soon feel asleep.[332]

Because the vicar slept until late the next day the sailors left without him. To his great astonishment he was told, upon entering the inn's dining-room for breakfast, that the boat he was to have sailed in had capsized early that morning and all of the men sailing in it had drowned.

Among reported paranormal experiences one of the most interesting involves a person hearing the voice of someone not physically present at the exact moment of their death or while they are experiencing some type of life-threatening crisis, a phenomenon referred to as a 'crisis apparition'.[333] In some instances the person whose voice was heard was at the time located in another city or even a different country to the hearer. The fact that the person had died or was undergoing a serious crisis at the time their voice was heard is sometimes only discovered much later. (The term *veridical* is sometimes used in regard to such experiences to indicate that, while they appear to involve auditory 'hallucinations', they nevertheless correspond to an actual external event, e.g. the death of a distant loved one). Such experiences are relatively common and are even occasionally reported in mainstream psychiatric literature, as in the following account which appeared in the *American Journal of Psychiatry*:

A 33-year old man described his experiences of his father's unexpected death while recuperating from surgery. Several days after the surgery the subject felt that his father 'came to him' while he was riding a bus and asked if he could leave because he was tired. The subject answered yes. Later he received a call from his brother saying that his father had died suddenly while apparently recovering excellently from the operation.[334]

Generally speaking the psychiatric profession has been curiously reluctant to attempt any serious investigation of paranormal phenomena. Nevertheless, there are some psychiatrists who have been sufficiently impressed by the available evidence to remain open-minded. Thus, in a 1983 article published in the *American Journal of Psychiatry*, Professor Ian Stevenson urged his colleagues not to automatically judge all 'hallucinations' to be pathological phenomena and to consider the possibility that *some* may involve paranormal aspects:

> Although persons who have unshared sensory experiences are often reluctant to tell others about them, many of them privately believe that their experiences include some extrasensory or paranormal communication. Most persons who believe this are probably mistaken; their experiences can often be explained fairly readily as due to coincidence, inference, faulty memory, or expectancy ... Also in the group of normally explicable hallucinations are those that occur when a person is falling asleep (hypnagogic) and awakening (hypnopompic). Nevertheless, after all such normal explanations have been considered, there remain some perceptual experiences that, upon careful investigation, do show evidence of extrasensory communication. But these experiences cannot be studied if the persons who have them are afraid to report them.[335]

An example of the phenomenon to which Professor Stevenson is referring involves what on one level might be called a 'bereavement hallucination' (this kind of experience, in which a deceased person's voice is heard by a surviving relative, was described in Chapter Two). Cases have been reported in which it appears that the voice of a deceased person conveyed information to the hearer which would not otherwise have been available to them. The highly respected Christian minister and author, John Sandford, has described such an experience:

> My mother purchased a used recliner chair. Having brought it home, she was cleaning it before use. While reaching deep between the cushion and the sidewall, she suddenly heard what she understood to be her mother's voice (several years after her death) saying, 'Reach deeper, Zelma.' She

did, and found an extremely valuable diamond ring, which the jeweller later sized to fit her. She wears it to this day, sure that it was a gift from her mother.[336]

Clinical experience has led some mental health professionals to give serious consideration to the possibility that a variety of apparently paranormal phenomena may sometimes occur in association with severe psychological and emotional disturbances.[337] For example, therapists who have worked closely with persons with Multiple Personality Disorder have noted and commented on the fact that alter personalities often appear to demonstrate ESP and other 'psychic' abilities.[338] One psychiatrist has even proposed the theory that schizophrenia may originate as a consequence of a person being continually overwhelmed by an influx of uncontrollable 'psychic impressions' or 'telepathic intrusions' which they are unable to screen out due to their extreme sensitivity.[339] While there has not yet been sufficient research to establish the validity of such theories there seems little doubt that people with a diagnosis of schizo-phrenia *do* occasionally demonstrate what seem to be true paranormal abilities mediated by voices. The following example was reported by a woman's treating psychiatrist:

> This was a woman who heard both higher- and lower-order voices. Her reclusive lifestyle in a small California town allowed her to live without anti-psychotic medications. The higher-order voices occasionally gave her tips on winning racehorses whenever she genuinely needed to supplement her meagre disability income. When she won, which she usually did, the lower-order voices would also try to give advice, but their predictions were invariably wrong. In fact, they usually picked the horse that came in last. She quickly learned to discriminate, and followed only the advice of the higher order.[340]

It should be noted that this same psychiatrist formed the opinion that *most* experiences of 'telepathy' among people with a diagnosis of schizophrenia seem to be the result of projections of their own fears or wishes. In most cases, he found, rather than having an ability to telepathically 'pick up' on what someone else is thinking the person is actually unconsciously attributing his or her *own* thoughts or wishes to others.

A growing number of mental health professionals acknowledge an interest in this realm (although such interests are often hidden in order to protect professional credibility). Thus, in a survey of psychiatrists and other medical doctors published in the *American Journal of Psychiatry* in 1980, 42% acknowledged that they believed in the possibility of 'psychic phenomena', while a further 35% stated that they had either had 'paranormal' experiences of some kind themselves or knew of someone who had.[341] In this context it is enlightening to learn about the views of some of the major figures in the history of psychiatry. For example, Sigmund Freud was highly sceptical about psychic phenomena for most of his life, unlike Carl Jung who always maintained a deep and abiding interest in the paranormal. He eventually became far less sceptical, however. Thus, in a footnote added to a later edition of one of his most important early books, *The Psychopathology of Everyday Life*, Freud said: 'I must however confess that in the last few years I have had a few remarkable experiences which might easily have been explained on the hypothesis of telepathic thought-transference.'[342] Freud wrote a number of important papers on the subjects of telepathy and the occult[343] and in 1911 joined the Society for Psychical Research. Toward the end of his life he had clearly developed a keen interest in parapsychological phenomena. Thus, in 1921 he said: 'I am not one of those who dismiss *a priori* the study of so-called occult psychic phenomena as unscientific, discreditable or even as dangerous. If I were at the beginning rather than at the end of a scientific career, as I am today, I might possibly choose just this field of research, in spite of all the difficulties.'[344]

10 *Spiritual Experiences*

As discussed in Chapter Two spiritual voice experiences of various kinds have been a significant source of comfort, reassurance, inspiration and guidance to people in every race and culture throughout human history. Indeed, in modern Western societies anyone who reports hearing voices *other* than in a religious or spiritual context is often likely to be treated with suspicion. By contrast, in many non-Western cultures it is taken for granted that a wide range of voice experiences have a supernatural origin, an assumption that was also made throughout Europe during the

Middle Ages. For example, in many parts of the world it would simply be assumed that anyone hearing the voice of a deceased person during bereavement had been in contact with the departed person's spirit. Likewise, it would be accepted that traditional healers such as shamans are empowered by their ability to contact, speak with and be guided by helping spirits.

People who have spiritual voice experiences may attribute them to various sources such as God, a Guardian Angel, the Inner Divine, the Spirit of Life, their own Higher Self, an Inner Guide or Teacher or simply to 'something greater than myself'. Whatever their ultimate origin there is no doubt that such voices invariably have a very profound impact on the hearer. Sometimes, as in the example cited below, the experience gives rise to feelings of deep inner peace and a greater sense of certainty about the ultimate meaning and purpose of life. However, even when the hearer experiences the voices as having a spiritual nature, he or she may still react with fear, doubt and confusion, especially during the initial stages of the revelation. Such reactions are especially likely if the hearer and others – including the culture as a whole – cling to rigid and negative views about voice experiences.

With the gradual re-awakening of interest in spirituality throughout highly materialistic Western societies during the past few decades has come a renewed interest among members of traditionally secular mental health professions in the possible spiritual origins of at least *some* types of voice experiences.[345] Under the influence of this nascent paradigm shift there are a growing number of clinicians who have come to believe that some severe psychological disturbances may have a significant spiritual dimension and be accompanied by voices which have a potentially healing influence. For example, psychology Professor David Lukoff has suggested that some disturbances which would ordinarily be classified as acute psychosis might be better understood as mystical experiences which have some psychosis-like aspects. He has referred to such states as 'mystical experiences with psychotic features'.[346] It is also possible, Professor Lukoff believes, that genuine spiritual experiences of various kinds may sometimes occur during the course of otherwise more mundane psychotic episodes (i.e. 'psychotic disorders with mystical features'). Voice experiences may also occur in the context of the type of transformational crisis that psychiatrist Stanislav Grof has termed a 'Spiritual Emergency'.[347] In the following example the profoundly healing effect of such a voice experience is clearly illustrated:

I will never forget one night in particular. I was in absolute terror, knowing I had to raise three children by myself. I cried all night. I thought I was losing my mind. I just couldn't gain control of myself ... At 11.00 am I went for a walk by myself down to the creek in the trees. I was still crying. I sat down on a rock. I knew I couldn't do everything I had to do in life with my limited self. Soon I heard a voice, an all-pervasive voice that seemed to be coming from everywhere. 'You are totally secure,' it said. The sound that came with it was the 'heavenly choir'. The message penetrated my whole being. I really got it. I began crying for joy. I was full of energy and floating on a cloud ... The *experience* was overwhelming and ecstatic! ... [it] was central in helping me become more relaxed about life and more trusting.[348]

As this example shows some voice experiences are accompanied by such a powerful sense of inner conviction and certainty that the hearer is left with absolutely no doubt about their spiritual origin. In other instances, however, a degree of uncertainty may be present. Some researchers have recently shown that, when the apparent power and authority of their 'omnipotent' voices was rigorously challenged, some people living with schizophrenia soon concluded that they had been mistaken about their supernatural nature.[349] The results of this type of research highlight the vital importance of applying a high level of spiritual discernment to voice experiences which appear to have a supernatural origin. Highly regarded spiritual authorities such as St Teresa of Avila and St John of the Cross (see Chapter Two) strongly emphasised the importance of rigorously applying discernment to voices (locutions) and urged anyone having such experiences to make every effort to determine whether they were of divine, demonic or imaginary origin.

Note: Some guidelines for the spiritual discernment of voices are provided in Chapter Seven.

11 *Spontaneous Self-Hypnosis*

The fact that people can sometimes be induced to hear voices as a result of hypnotic suggestion was discussed in Chapter One. Charles Tart, a psychologist who has intensively investigated altered states of consciousness, has described the relative ease with which hypnosis can be used to create a vivid sensory impression of the voice of an apparently independent entity:

> From my studies with hypnosis I know I can set up an apparently independent existent entity whose characteristics are constructed to my specifications and the person hypnotised will experience it as if it's something outside of his own consciousness talking.[350]

A number of investigators have suggested that, when severely stressed or threatened, some people may attempt to protect themselves by spontaneously withdrawing into a trance state which they *unconsciously* induce using self-hypnosis. In the ensuing altered state of consciousness voices and other unusual experiences may occur:

> A hypnotic potential for hallucinations has been known since the time of Mesmer. What has not been recognised is the tendency of some excellent hypnotic subjects to enter spontaneous trances where voices, visions, delusions, and personalities can be hypnotically, but unknowingly, generated by the subject himself. Often these voices and delusions may then operate even when the individual is in an alert state. The mental mechanisms responsible for auditory hallucinations are controversial. Only one explanation at present can be both experimentally and clinically verified, and that is hypnosis. Many excellent hypnotic subjects in a trance, either induced by a hypnotist of spontaneously engendered, can hear with realism various sounds or voices . . . [351]

Some investigators believe that spontaneous self-hypnosis may be one of the major factors contributing to the development of Multiple Personality Disorder. According to this view MPD occurs as a result of a person's *unrecognised* use of self-hypnosis to create personalities beginning at a very early age (usually between 4 and 6 years). Using self-hypnosis in this way enables a severely traumatised child to delegate experiences or functions to one or more 'alter' personalities while the amnesia of hypnosis leaves the abuse victim unaware of their existence.[352] It should be noted that even if MPD could be accounted for on the basis of hypnotically-generated personalities it remains unclear to what extent (if any) spontaneous self-hypnosis might play a part in the origin of voices in people without MPD. It is interesting to note, however, that in one study of people who reported hearing voices (most of whom had been given a diagnosis of schizophrenia), 60% turned out to have 'alter' personalities responsible for the voices.[353] It is also noteworthy that people who had imaginary companions in childhood appear to be better hypnotic subjects than those who had none.[354]

12 The Theory of the Bicameral Mind

Princeton University psychology professor Julian Jaynes has developed a novel hypothesis to account for voice experiences based on his extensive research into the nature and origins of human consciousness.[355] Jaynes believes that consciousness is a relatively new phenomenon which human beings did not possess until quite late in their evolutionary history. Before about 2000 BC humans lacked conscious self-awareness and were consequently incapable of making decisions on the basis of rational thought since to do so requires conscious processes (e.g. thinking about a situation, considering possible alternative courses of action, considering future consequences, making a decision, then acting). Since early human beings were capable of carrying out complex patterns of behaviour even though they lacked consciousness some other means of decision-making must have been available to them. Jaynes believes that this occurred through the medium of voices. In ancient times, he suggests, the first steps in making a decision involved a communication process which took place within the bicameral (literally, 'two chambered') mind. Thus, a command to act in a certain way would arise in the right hemisphere of the brain and be coded into a 'voice' which was then 'heard' by the left hemisphere and obediently acted upon. Whenever a decision had to be made a voice would be heard:

During the eras of the bicameral mind, we may suppose that the stress threshold for hallucinations was much, much lower than in either normal people or schizophrenics today. The only stress necessary was that which occurs when a change in behaviour is necessary because of some novelty in a situation. Anything that could not be dealt with on the basis of habit, any conflict between work and fatigue, between attack and flight, any choice between whom to obey or what to do, anything that required any decision at all was sufficient to cause an auditory hallucination.[356]

Jaynes believes that the admonitory voices were usually attributed to gods. By about 500 BC human beings had evolved to the point of being capable of conscious decision-making and so the 'guiding voice' of earlier times was gradually replaced by rational thought processes. Jaynes has suggested that the reason voice experiences are still common today is related to the fact that in evolutionary terms they once served an essential function. Indeed, he has gone as far as to suggest that if the experience of hearing voices is taken to be a psychotic symptom, then it could be said that before the second millennium BC *every* human being was schizophrenic![357]

13 *Information Processing Dysfunction*

Some psychologists have attempted to explain the voice experiences associated with schizophrenia in terms of the existence of abnormalities or disturbances in the way the hearer's mind processes information.[358] Generally speaking these theories are based on the assumption that at any given moment there are a vast number of mental processes going on within the mind that remain totally unconscious (i.e. they occur outside of awareness). In very simple terms this might be compared to the fact that, while there are many complex electronic processes constantly occurring in a radio, all we are usually aware of is the sound which finally emanates from it. In a similar way, although a wide variety of thoughts, memories, feelings and wishes are constantly occurring within a person's mind, most of this mental activity normally remains outside of their awareness. Some researchers have hypothesised that people with a diagnosis of schizophrenia may hear voices as a result of some kind of 'leakage' or 'spilling over' into awareness of aspects of mental activity which would ordinarily remain unconscious.[359] It has been suggested that one reason this occurs may be related to some type of failure or breakdown of the automatic mechanisms in the mind that ordinarily filter out of awareness most mental activity. According to this view such a breakdown in 'perceptual filtering' could result in a person becoming hyper-aware of internally generated thoughts and images which may then be experienced as voices which seem to emanate from outside the hearer's mind. Norma MacDonald has given the following account of a 'breakdown in perceptual filtering' which she believes was at the core of her own experience of schizophrenia:

> Each of us is capable of coping with a large number of stimuli, invading our being through any of the senses. [However] we would be incapable of carrying on any of our daily activities if even one-hundredth of all these available stimuli invaded us at once. So the mind must have a filter which functions without our conscious thought, sorting stimuli and allowing only those which are relevant to the situation in hand to disturb consciousness. And this filter must be working at maximum efficiency at all times, particularly when we require a high degree of concentration. What happened to me ... was a breakdown in the filter, and a hodge-podge of unrelated stimuli were distracting me from things which should have had my undivided attention ... I had very little ability to sort the relevant from the irrelevant. The filter had broken down. Completely unrelated events became intricately connected in my mind.[360]

The fact that people living with schizophrenia are often most likely to hear voices when they are experiencing high levels of *internal* emotional arousal (e.g. stress, anxiety) combined with low levels of *external* auditory input (e.g. isolation, sensory under-stimulation) has been interpreted as lending support to the information-processing theory of voices.[361]

14 *Biomedical Theories*

Within the purview of the so-called 'medical model' voice experiences of various kinds are usually grouped together and classified as auditory hallucinations (i.e. 'false sensory perceptions'). Such voices are frequently considered to be psychotic symptoms and are thus often regarded as being symptomatic of schizophrenia (see Chapter Three). Psychiatrists who adhere to the biomedical approach refer to hallucinations and delusions as 'positive' psychotic symptoms and allege that they are associated with – if not specifically caused by – a 'chemical imbalance' or some other kind of abnormality in the diagnosed person's brain. In keeping with these views it has been suggested by one well-known author that the voices of schizophrenia are a direct result of the way in which 'the schizophrenic disease process selectively affects the auditory tract or auditory centers in the brain, thereby producing auditory hallucinations'.[362] In recent years researchers have used highly sophisticated brain imaging techniques in an effort to locate the specific functional and structural abnormalities which are considered to be responsible for causing voices.[363] The belief that a 'chemical imbalance' in the brain is responsible for voices and other psychotic symptoms provides the rationale for the use of neuroleptic medications since these drugs are believed to selectively block the post-synaptic receptors for dopamine, a neurotransmitter widely thought to be associated with schizophrenia.

Attempts to account for voices in purely biological terms have yet to adequately address the complex 'chicken and egg' question regarding the direction of any link that may exist between physical changes in the brain and the onset of the voices (i.e. are voices caused by changes in the brain or do alterations in brain functioning merely reflect the occurrence of voice experiences?). In this regard it is important to note that recent research has established that a person's subjective experiences can result in neurochemical and neuroanatomical changes in their brain.[364] Biological theories of voices also leave unanswered the question of why the specific experiences of people vary so much from one individual to another. For example, if every person who receives a diagnosis of schizophrenia has some kind of genetically-inherited 'chemical imbalance' in their brain which is solely responsible for causing their symptoms, how is it that some hear harsh persecutory or critical voices while others hear voices which are friendly and supportive (and many hear a mixture of both)? Some psychiatrists have attempted to answer this question by suggesting that some kind of disturbance in the diagnosed person's brain may be responsible for causing the voices to occur in the first place, but that their specific individualised *content* (i.e. who the voices seem to be and what they say) is primarily determined by factors which are closely related to the hearer's psychological make-up and social circumstances.[365] In line with this approach it has been suggested that psychological and social factors may determine the content of voices in a similar manner to what occurs in dreams:

> The content of hallucinations in 'functional psychoses' seems most clearly related to previous life experience. In this sense, hallucinations during the waking state and those during dreams are probably quite similar, as Freud suggested. Those whose vulnerability is stressed and who are afraid of injury will hallucinate that they are under attack, while those whose vulnerability is stressed and have unresolved feelings of guilt will be told that they are 'sinners'. The content of the 'voices' . . . relates to the general psychodynamics and the specific fears and wishes of the individual.[366]

Currently the two most influential views regarding the aetiology (causation) of the voices of schizophrenia are those derived from biological psychiatry and those based on variations of the concept of an underlying information processing dysfunction (models involving some combination of these two views are also possible). It is widely acknowledged that neither of these two schools of thought (or various combinations of them) are able to provide an entirely satisfactory or truly comprehensive account of hallucinatory voices or the other positive symptoms of schizophrenia.[367] Furthermore, it is unclear what relevance these theories might have to voice experiences which occur outside the context of schizophrenia or other kinds of 'mental illness'. It seems extremely unlikely that they could account for the extraordinarily wide variety of voice experiences that are described in this book, including those experienced by many members of the so-called 'normal' population, those which have a genuine and uplifting spiritual nature, and those which exert a positive and creative influence on the hearer's life. In view of these limitations some psychiatrists have argued that priority should be given to expanding the psychiatric perspective beyond biology in order to develop an approach to voices which incorporates a wider range of the many factors now known to be relevant to their occurrence.[368]

Conclusion

It is clear that voices are not merely something that happens in the hearer's brain, nor do they occur in a psychological, social and spiritual vacuum. Rather, hearing voices is an *experience* which is had by a human being. As such it occurs within the context of a particular personality structure and physiological constitution, a specific set of psychological, social and cultural circumstances, and under the influence of various personal and transpersonal spiritual imperatives. Since human beings and their inner experiences are both complex and multi-faceted no attempt to account for voices can be complete unless it is genuinely *holistic*. In other words, all of the relevant psychological, social, spiritual and biological factors must be taken into consideration if the true nature and origin of voice experiences is to be understood.

Seeking a viable explanation for voices (whether one's own or those of other people) is not simply an intellectual exercise or a matter of theoretical interest – although it undoubtedly *is* both of these things since the phenomenon of voices raises many important and challenging questions regarding the structure of the human personality, the nature of mind, and the ontological status of spiritual and paranormal phenomena. This particular quest has, in addition, a number of important *practical* ramifications. What a person believes about the nature and origin of voices will strongly influence how they respond to them. Thus, if voices are viewed as 'auditory hallucinations' caused by some kind of 'chemical imbalance', neuroleptic drugs may be seen as a valid and appropriate way of dealing with them, the aim being to eliminate them as quickly as possible. On the other hand, if the voices are believed to have significant psychological roots or an important spiritual dimension, it may be more useful to accept and listen to them or seek ways to work with them therapeutically. Rather than attempting to understand or 'explain' their voices some people may be content to take a very pragmatic approach which involves exploring ways of learning to live with them more comfortably or developing practical coping strategies which help them to achieve or maintain a greater sense of control.

Anyone who delves into the complexities of voice experiences will very quickly discover that, despite the advent of modern 'high tech' approaches to the brain and the development and refinement of sophisticated psychological theories, our understanding of these phenomena remains extremely limited. It is sobering to realise how profoundly ignorant we are about the ultimate nature and purpose of *many* aspects of human experiencing. Intelligence, creativity, spirituality, dreams, fantasy and love are but a few of the many possible examples of areas which continue to be enigmatic. Carl Jung was very much of the opinion that there are certain aspects of life – and of the psyche in particular – which will always remain a mystery to human beings. It is humbling to realise that this is probably also true of many kinds of voice experiences.

Chapter Seven

A REALM OF SPIRITS?

*All cultures, including our own, acknowledge the existence
of spirits at levels beyond the human. We call them angels,
but they go under different names in other traditions. This is
one of the most fundamental themes in human spiritual and
religious experience.*

– Fox and Sheldrake[369]

People who hear voices sometimes attribute them to spirits, angels, gods, or supernatural guides of one kind or another. In modern Western societies such ideas are frequently looked upon as mere superstitions which belong to a 'primitive' and pre-scientific era, and the experiences which give rise to them are often summarily dismissed as being the products of an overactive or excessively vivid imagination – if they are not judged to be the hallucinations of a seriously disturbed psychotic mind. In spite of such negative attitudes experiences which are claimed to involve contact with spirits are relatively common and occur in a wide variety of circumstances, as previous chapters have shown. Such claims raise the question of whether there could really be such things as 'spirits' and, if there are, what their true nature and origin might be.

According to the Oxford Dictionary a spirit is a 'supernatural, incorporeal, rational being or personality, usually regarded as imperceptible at ordinary times to the human senses, but capable of becoming visible at pleasure, and frequently conceived as troublesome, terrifying or hostile to mankind.' This definition emphasises the fact that, while they are ordinarily invisible to human beings, spirits are capable of making their presence felt if they so choose. This ability gives them considerable power and is one of the reasons they are always treated with the greatest respect by those who take them to be real. Whether or not spirits are in fact autonomous supernatural beings it is clear that many people who believe in them have experienced *something* which appears to extend beyond the usual boundaries of everyday physical existence. Such experiences, whether they are felt to be positive or negative, are often profoundly moving and may sometimes even be life-changing in their impact.

Readers who are prepared to put aside any preconceptions they might have in order to consider this issue with an open mind will soon discover that, whatever 'spirits' may happen to be in reality, experiences which purportedly involve them have played a significant role in the lives of human beings in every part of the world throughout recorded history. Although there exists a powerful cultural taboo which tends to silence discussion of this subject (particularly in academic and professional circles), an unbiased examination of this whole realm of human experience is essential to the task of developing a truly comprehensive understanding of voices. The aim of this chapter is to provide a broad over-view of a range of different perspectives relevant to the phenomenon of 'spirits' and to offer some suggestions regarding what its connection might be to the experience of hearing voices.

Spirits in the Christian Tradition

In the Christian tradition non-physical supernatural beings are accepted as a reality and a universal part of human experience. In the New Testament numerous references are made to the existence of three types of such non-physical entities or beings: angels, spirits and demons. *Angels* derive their name from the Greek word for 'messenger' and their appearances and the various missions they performed among human beings are referred to 74 times in the Gospels and Acts. Angels can be from either God or Satan although unless stated otherwise they are usually assumed to be good spiritual messengers who act as representatives of God. *Spirits* are described as independent, non-physical beings on somewhat the same level as humans but of a lower spiritual order than the angels or demons. They are capable of knowing, desiring, and acting and can be subject either to God or Satan, to other spiritual realities, or even to men and women. Malicious spirits are described in the New Testament as being demonic, unclean, evil, and capable of causing infirmity. *Demons* are spirit beings, either good or bad, which are inferior to God but superior to human beings. Most of the New Testament references to demons concern malignant entities and instances of demonic possession are described 13 times in the Gospels.[370] Traditional Christian teaching places great emphasis on the reality and importance of the spirit-world and the relationship that exists between it, material reality and the world of human beings:

> The New Testament [gives] a very clear picture of two worlds which impinge upon each other. There is a world of matter and also a world of spiritual reality which includes God, the devil, angels, demons, both good and evil (unclean) spirits, principalities, thrones, powers, dominions, authorities, and beggarly elements. The human being is caught between these two worlds and participates in both of them. This second realm, in which the human being experiences realities equally as important as matter, is met in dreams, visions, and spiritual encounters of various kinds. Even when people are not aware of this world, the beings in it influence them ... [371]

The belief that supernatural beings are real and can have a significant influence on human affairs has been accepted by many highly respected Christian teachers. For example, St Thomas Aquinas (1225–1274), a Dominican monk widely acknowledged to be one of the greatest of all Catholic theologians, is also known as 'Doctor Angelicus' (the angelic doctor) because he studied and wrote extensively on the subject of angels. Aquinas believed that, among their other roles, angels have the important task of carrying divine revelations and spiritual enlightenment to human beings.[372]

Helping and Guiding Spirits

When faced with circumstances involving extreme emotional or physical distress (especially when combined with prolonged isolation) some people have reported having unexpected encounters with what they felt were helping or guiding 'spirits'. A graphic account of such an experience was provided by Captain Joshua Slocum, the first sailor to circumnavigate the world single-handedly. While sailing his yacht alone at the turn of the century he endured conditions of extreme physical stress and profound isolation. In his account of this epic voyage Slocum tells how at one especially difficult point in the journey he became sick during a gale and had retired below decks to rest. All of a sudden a 'phantom' helmsman appeared and took the helm:

> Then I went below, and threw myself upon the cabin floor in great pain. How long I lay there I could not tell, for I became delirious. When I came to, as I thought, from my swoon, I realised that the sloop was plunging into a heavy sea, and looking out of the companionway, to my amazement I saw a tall man at the helm. His rigid hand, grasping the spokes of the wheel, held them as in a vice. One may imagine my astonishment. His rig was that of a foreign sailor, and the large red cap he wore was cockbilled over his left ear, and all was set off with shaggy black whiskers. He would have been taken for a pirate in any part of the world. While I gazed upon his threatening aspect I forgot the storm, and wondered if he had come to cut my throat. This he seemed to divine. 'Señor', said he, doffing his cap, 'I have come to do you no harm ... I am one of Columbus's crew,' he continued. 'I am the pilot of the *Pinta* come to aid you. Lie quiet, señor captain,' he added, 'and I will guide your ship tonight.'[373]

To his astonishment Captain Slocum discovered the next morning that his boat was still heading on the exact course he had put it on before he became sick and that it had covered ninety miles during the night through a rough sea. The phantom pilot reappeared in a dream the next night and said he would return whenever he was needed. Slocum says he woke refreshed with the feeling that he had been in the presence of 'a friend and a seaman of vast experience'. Over the next three years the phantom reappeared several times during gales.

Throughout history there have been numerous reports of encounters with what some people believe are 'helping spirits' or 'guardian angels'. In recent years, for example, many people who have had a near-death experience (NDE) have described meeting and being guided by a benevolent spirit presence (NDEs were discussed in Chapter One). There have also been many reports (some made by hospital nurses and doctors) of persons on the point of death being visited by an angel or the spirit of some long-deceased family member who has come to help them make their crossing to the 'other side'. Interestingly, people often appear to change visibly following such an encounter, with many becoming elated and expressing their readiness to depart from this world.[374]

In contrast to those who experience a spontaneous one-off encounter with a 'helping spirit' during a crisis situation, certain individuals such as shamans and spiritualist mediums deliberately seek and cultivate a long-term relationship with one or more helping spirit and rely upon them for wisdom and guidance (see below).

The Spirits of Shamanism

Spirits of various kinds are accepted as an integral aspect of reality in many non-Western cultures. Such spirits are believed to be present throughout the natural world and to dwell in water, air, earth and fire as well as in animals and plants. These spirits, powerful and ever-present, are considered to be capable of affecting the lives of human beings in many ways. It is widely believed, for example, that good or bad events, fortunate or unfortunate circumstances, and success or failure in various undertakings can all be influenced in one way or another by spirits. Consequently, ritual offerings are often made and various ceremonial acts performed in an effort to please or placate them. In many societies dreams, deliberately induced trance-states, and various forms of *benign* possession* are among the wide range of techniques that are specifically employed to foster awareness of and communication with the spirit-world.[375] Shamans are often very important figures within such cultures since it is they alone who are capable of actually controlling the spirits.

The central role played by tutelary spirits in the lives of shamans was described in Chapter Two. To become a 'master of spirits' a shaman must learn to control a number of spirits. Those he does control become the helping spirits which assist him by teaching, instructing and providing the strength and ability required

---

*People often tend to think of possession only in *negative* terms (e.g. possession by malevolent or demonic influences). However, it is important to understand that possession states can also be a positive phenomenon. Christians value possession by the Holy Spirit, for example, and in many non-Western cultures various spirits, deities and gods may be invoked and invited to possess persons participating in healing rituals or ceremonial worship. The term *benign* indicates that the state is in some way beneficial to the individual concerned.

to fulfil his roles of healing and guiding. Shamans have immediate and concrete experience with their helping spirits: they see and talk with them as if with ordinary people and often develop an intensely personal and intimate relationship with them:

> A healer's relationship with his helping spirit is often no different from his relationship with his fellow beings. It frequently resembles a marriage and displays the whole spectrum of human emotions such as love, hate, jealousy, distrust, obedience, fear, longing, quarrels, etc. This is difficult to understand for those who had no imaginary friends when they were children or who never encountered helping spirits in an extreme state of exhaustion.[376]

It is very important to emphasise that even in cultures in which shamanism is an accepted practice a clear distinction is nevertheless made between those who have learnt to control and work with spirits (shamans are acknowledged to be 'masters of spirits') and those who, for one reason or another, appear to have become a mere 'plaything' of the spirit-world. The following anecdote clearly illustrates this crucial difference:

> The ability to enter into and exit from ecstatic states of consciousness and the spirit world at will is one characteristic that distinguishes shamans from the mentally ill. For example, [the anthropologist] Michael Harner reported that, 'When I was with the Jivaro or Shuar tribe, there was a man who wandered the forest day and night talking to spirits. So I asked if this man were a shaman. 'No', they said, 'he's crazy.' Was he crazy because he was seeing things? No, because they had seen them too. He was crazy because he was out of control – he couldn't turn it off.'[377]

The Shamanic Initiatory Crisis

As explained above, a belief in spirits and the role of shamans in communicating with them is an integral part of the cultural tradition of many non-Western societies. There is growing evidence that people in Western societies, too, may sometimes have experiences which bear a striking similarity to those of traditional shamans. The psychiatrist Stanislav Grof believes that as part of what he terms a

'Spiritual Emergency' some people undergo a profound psychospiritual transformation which involves spontaneous experiences closely resembling those of the shamanic initiatory crisis ('shamanic illness') described in Chapter Two.[378] Persons undergoing such a crisis experience a journey into the underworld ('the realm of the dead') where they undergo a series of terrifying ordeals culminating in a symbolic death and rebirth. Following this process of initiation some persons may continue to experience the presence of various deities, spirit guides or power animals from whom teachings and guidance are received.

The experiences of David Lukoff provide a graphic illustration of this type of uninvited encounter with 'spirits'. Lukoff, now an American psychology professor, had a psychotic episode at the age of twenty-three which turned out to be a profound initiatory experience. Having dropped out of a doctoral programme in anthropology, he was hitchhiking around the country and experimenting with psychedelic drugs as part of his search for the 'meaning of life'. One day he had the sudden, life-changing revelation that the journal he had been keeping as part of his daily routine was to become a 'new Bible'. Believing that it was his personal mission to write and disseminate a new 'holy book' that would unite the world and create an international society free of conflict and full of love Lukoff felt himself to be inspired by direct contact with guiding spirits:

> While writing my 'new Bible' I held internal conversations with the 'spirits' of eminent thinkers in the social sciences and humanities. I had discussions with contemporary persons, including R.D. Laing, Margaret Mead, and Bob Dylan, as well as individuals no longer living, such as Rousseau, Freud, Jung, and – of course – Buddha and Christ. I talked with them about the design of a new society that would herald a return to tribal living and I recorded brief summaries of the 'messages' I obtained from each of them. While writing, the apparent clarity of my thoughts and beauty of my vision sometimes brought tears to my eyes. After initially assuming 'The Scholar' as a pen name alluding to the erudite origins of this project, I soon adopted 'The Scholar' as my new reincarnated identity. In five days I produced a forty-seven-page book that contained a

combination of parables, poems, and instructions for organising the new society.[379]

Sadly, over the next year he gradually began to realise that his 'new Bible' was in reality nothing more than a semi-coherent collection of unoriginal ideas. Filled with embarrassment and mourning the loss of the mission that had once filled his life with great meaning and purpose, he began to contemplate suicide. However, his life was once again to change quite unexpectedly:

> The book had been my raison d'etre for the previous several months, and now it seemed worthless. I felt totally lost and confused . . . I began to consider the possibility of committing suicide. The image of my skeleton spontaneously appeared to me on several sleepless nights. During the height of these difficulties I went for a walk near the bay, ruminating about events of the last six months. Suddenly I heard a voice say, 'Become a healer'. I was startled. At that time, lost in self-recrimination, I didn't even think of myself as having a future. However, this voice – the only disembodied voice I've ever heard emanate from outside of myself – set a whole new sequence of events in motion. Prior to this episode the healing arts had never interested me. Yet this voice set me on the path towards my own healing – and a new career.[380]

For several years after he received this vocational call Lukoff involved himself intensively in the study of a wide range of holistic healing practices. In his opinion the true spiritual potential of his 'psychotic' experience remained dormant until nine years later when he began studying shamanism. Contact with shamans helped to reassure him of his sanity, he has said, particularly as he was told by one highly respected Cheyenne medicine man that his temporary psychosis had been brought on by spirits in order to communicate teachings.

Spiritualism and Channelling

During the first year of bereavement – and often for very much longer thereafter – many people feel the presence of, see, or hear the voice of (and sometimes even speak with) the deceased person.

Although in Western societies these surprisingly common experiences are likely to be considered a type of 'bereavement hallucination', people in traditional non-Western cultures often consider them to be instances of contact with the spirit of the deceased person.

For at least the past one hundred and fifty years adherents of spiritualism have claimed that certain people possess the ability to deliberately make contact with the spirits of deceased human beings. Such people, who are commonly known as 'mediums', often claim that they are able to speak with these spirits and relay their spoken replies to questions put to them (by the participants in a seance, for example). Many mediums rely upon a personal protecting spirit (a so-called 'spirit control') to help them make contact with other spirits with whom the medium has no personal connection. In this respect 'spirit controls' serve a similar function for a medium as do the 'helping spirits' of the shaman.

At the present time scientifically acceptable evidence supporting the claims of spiritualism is lacking. In spite of this there are some mediums who have gained considerable reputations as a result of the accuracy of the information they have allegedly been able to obtain from spirits. There are undoubtedly some cases in which a medium (now often called a 'channel' since contemporary mediumship is often referred to as channelling) appears to obtain information or develops abilities for which no mundane explanation is readily available. A possible example of this can be found in the case of Rosemary Brown, a London housewife who claims to have held 'spirit conversations' with the classical composer Franz Liszt who died in 1886. Brown claims that Liszt has dictated musical compositions to her and introduced her to the spirits of Beethoven, Chopin, Schubert, Brahms and Debussy, all of whom also transmitted new musical works to her. A recording of these 'spirit' compositions has been acclaimed by highly regarded professional music critics who have been impressed by their faithfulness to the style of the original composers.[381] Rosemary Brown has subsequently written a book in which she provides detailed reports of her conversations with the 'spirits' of a number of deceased eminent people including the genius physicist Albert Einstein and the philosopher Bertrand Russell.[382]

Interestingly, people who develop mediumistic abilities often describe having had vivid experiences with imaginary companions since early childhood. For example, the famous medium Doris Stokes has told of the 'spirit children' who became her secret companions when she was only six or seven years old.[383]

Spirits and Psychiatric Disorder

Many people who have experienced severe psychological disturbances ('mental illness') of various kinds feel that they have come into direct contact with supernatural beings at some point during their ordeals. Persons with multiple personality disorder (MPD), for example, often report having 'alters' which they variously identify as spirit guides, astral entities, spirits of the dead, or even demons. Some MPD therapists have even conducted exorcisms in specific cases in an effort to banish malevolent persecutor alter personalities.[384] People experiencing psychosis – schizophrenia in particular – frequently attribute their voices to supernatural beings (see Chapter Four). Indeed, the earliest theories about the causes of madness were based on the belief that the disturbed person was possessed by a supernatural entity, a view which still prevails in many non-Western cultures. The experience of hearing voices undoubtedly contributes to this idea, as Jung has explained:

> There can be no doubt that mental illnesses play a significant part in causing belief in spirits ... In all ages and all over the world, insane people have been regarded as possessed by evil spirits, and this belief is supported by the patients own hallucinations. The patients are tormented less by visions than by auditory hallucinations: they hear 'voices'. Very often these voices are those of relatives or of persons in some way connected with the patient's conflicts. To the naïve mind, the hallucinations naturally appear to be caused by spirits.[385]

The following anecdote, written by a person with a diagnosis of schizophrenia, illustrates Jung's point and clearly highlights the dilemma that is faced by many persons who experience severe mental disturbances in which voices are a prominent feature:

> An uninitiated person would probably be very much startled over such phenomena. For example, what would

you think if you were on a level, desolate tract of land without any vegetation, or places of concealment upon it, and without a human being within miles, you heard a mysterious, seemingly unearthly voice answer a question you were just thinking about? Maybe you would think you were listening to a spirit voice. Or would you think it were the voice of an angel? Maybe you would think that the Holy Ghost, or God was speaking to you. Suppose the voice said: 'I am God', and then ordered you to do various things. Would you do as the voice directed, even if it cost you your life? Some persons would.[386]

A belief in the reality of spirits and their ability to interact with and influence the behaviour of human beings is an accepted part of the normal world view of many traditional cultures. Consequently, disturbed persons who are considered to be under their influence are often treated with appropriate culturally-sanctioned methods such as healing rituals conducted by shamans. Psychiatric anthropologists who have studied these approaches have often been impressed by their apparent effectiveness.[387] By contemporary Western medical standards such approaches are often considered to be unscientific – if not primitive. Nevertheless, there are some conventionally trained mental health professionals whose research has led them to very different conclusions regarding the origin and nature of some of the voice experiences which occur in the context of severe mental disturbance.

Using a technique similar to one employed by MPD therapists the clinical psychologist Wilson Van Dusen found that it was possible to talk with the voices of many of his patients.[388] This discovery led him to conduct an intensive study of the inner experience of hallucinations over the course of seventeen years working in psychiatric hospitals. He found that most patients had similar experiences despite having received a wide variety of different diagnoses. After many years of investigation Van Dusen reached the rather surprising conclusion that many of his patients' voice experiences appeared to be the result of their interaction with a realm of spirits. He found that these spirits could be divided according to their nature into a benevolent 'higher' and a malevolent 'lower' order. Some people seem to hear only voices of the lower order while others experience both kinds.

Van Dusen found that voices belonging to the lower order

are predominantly persecutory. They invariably act against the person's will and are persistently attacking and malevolent. They often talk a lot but always have a limited vocabulary and range of concerns (e.g. they sometimes endlessly repeat a few ideas or simple statements – one man's voice simply said 'hey' for months on end). These voices use trickery to deceive the hearer as to their powers and will threaten, cajole, entreat, and attempt to undermine in every conceivable way (e.g. they may offer helpful sounding advice only to catch the person out in some weakness). Since they always see only the negative side of everything nothing pleases them. Van Dusen concluded that their general aim seems to be to take over the hearer and live through them as they please. In order to do this they will lie, cheat, deceive, pretend and threaten:

> Lower order voices are as though one is dealing with drunken bums at a bar who like to tease and torment just for the fun of it. They will suggest lewd acts and then scold the patient for considering them. They find a weak point of conscience and work on it interminably. For instance, one man heard voices teasing him for three years over a ten-cent debt he had already paid. They call the patient every conceivable name, suggest every lewd act, steal memories or ideas right out of consciousness, threaten death, and work on the patient's credibility in every way. For instance they will brag that they will produce some disaster on the morrow and then claim some honour for one in the daily papers. They suggest foolish acts (such as: Raise your right hand in the air and stay that way) and tease if he does it and threaten if he doesn't ... Many patients have heard loud and clear voices plotting their death for weeks on end ... They threaten pain and can cause felt pain as a way of enforcing their power. The most devastating experience of all is to be shouted at constantly by dozens of voices ... They invade every nook and cranny of privacy, work on every weakness and credibility, claim awesome powers, lie, make promises and then undermine the patient's will.[389]

Lower order voices have less knowledge and talent than the hearer and, while they never have their own personal identity, will often accept any name and identity they are given (e.g. when identified as some person known to the hearer they are able to assume that person's voice quality perfectly). However, the voice quality may then change so that it sounds like someone else, thus leaving the hearer totally confused as to who is actually speaking. Voices of the lower order are invariably irreligious and some are so vehemently anti-religious that they will actively attempt to interfere with the hearer's religious or spiritual practices. Van Dusen was struck by the similarity of lower order voice experiences to medieval accounts of possession. Given their often extremely malicious nature it is little wonder that many psychiatric patients with lower order voices do indeed become convinced that they are possessed by evil spirits.[390] (In this regard it is interesting to note that some psychiatrists have observed people recovering from acute psychotic episodes who have been beset by threatening voices after they dabbled in occult practices such as experimenting with Ouija boards or attempting to conduct seances.[391])

Although apparently much less common (accounting for about one quarter or less of his patient's experiences), higher order hallucinations appear to be just the opposite of the lower order.* Van Dusen likened them to 'angels' which had come to help the person. Like wise and considerate instructors the higher order is invariably more gifted and creative than the hearer and always acts out of great respect and concern for their welfare. Interestingly, they are often non-verbal (some don't speak at all and are purely visual) and are experienced as being more internal, feeling-related and subtle. They seem to communicate directly with the person's inner feelings and motives, often in a highly symbolic and religious way which is emotionally very powerful and carries 'an almost inexpressible ring of truth'. The intensely radiant presence of some 'Christ-like figures' from the higher order may have the effect of leading the person to a greater understanding of his or her inner potentials. The higher order seem to be extremely intuitive regarding the person or anyone else present and often seem to have extrasensory powers. Van Dusen was particularly impressed by the

---

*Van Dusen has suggested that the apparent rarity of the higher order may be related to the fact that these experiences are often extremely subtle, frequently non-verbal, and tend to be directed to the person's inner life. Because their presence is not so obvious they are only rarely reported.

extraordinary wisdom they often seem to possess. He discovered, for example, that some poorly educated and unsophisticated people (some had even been lifelong criminals) heard spiritually elevated higher order voices. One voice, a woman who referred to herself as 'An Emanation of the Feminine Aspect of the Divine', was the most gifted person in the area of religion Van Dusen had ever encountered:

> She was the hallucination in the head of a high school-educated, schizophrenic, not very gifted gas pipefitter ... He had mean critical voices working at him and she came to cheer him up ... He described her as a most pleasant companion. I first sensed her gift in the form of all the universal symbols she produced. They came so fast that few of them could be described ... Some seemed to pertain to ancient myths. I went home and studied some obscure part of Greek myths and asked her about it the next time I saw the gas pipefitter. She not only understood the myth, she saw its human implications better than I did ... The more serious and deep a question, the more depth in her answer. She was entirely unlike talking to earthly theologians who call on history or doctrine to prove a point. She knew the depth of my understanding and led gently into very human allusions that reflected a profound understanding of history ... The patient didn't understand my conversations with her. He had no religious interests. I remember once his turning in the doorway as he was leaving and asking me to give him a clue as to what she and I had just talked about.[392]

Experiences such as this convinced Van Dusen that psychiatric patients may sometimes be shown things of great importance in their hallucinations. He concluded, for example, that voices may sometimes reflect the person's unrecognised, unlived-out potentials: the higher order reflect creative talents and unused gifts while the lower order illustrate personal faults, blindness and stupidity (the higher order itself explained that the function of the lower order was basically to illustrate and make conscious the hearer's weaknesses and faults). Unfortunately, people are often unable to understand or make full creative use of such voice experiences due to the fact that, as with dreams, their communications are usually highly symbolic and are therefore readily open to misunderstanding and misinterpretation.

What are 'Spirits'?

Many religious and cultural groups and large numbers of individuals believe in the existence of spirits. However, across this broad spectrum there are many very different views concerning their precise nature. For example, there are those who simply accept spirits as independent supernatural beings which have the capacity to influence human beings for good or ill. On the other hand, some people think of spirits not as literal beings but more as personified energies or forces which can influence human thoughts, feelings and behaviour. In this view a spirit might be understood as the active or essential power of some emotion or mental state. In line with this understanding, 'devils' or 'demons' have been construed as personifications of weaknesses or other undesirable traits or tendencies. For example, the well known 'seven deadly sins' involve undesirable passions (Lust, Greed, Gluttony), destructive emotions (Anger, Pride, Envy), and negative behaviours (Laziness), and are sometimes attributed to the influence of malign spirits (for example, the spirits of envy, greed, pride and so on). According to this view, rather than coming from *outside* a person, spirits and demons arise from tendencies or characteristics that exist *within* them.

The question of whether spirits are generated from within a person or if they actually are independently existing supernatural entities is a topic which has generated much debate among theologians, psychologists, anthropologists and others over many centuries. In the end, anyone who has had experiences that seem to be related to spirits must make up their own mind about what to believe. Those who accept a particular religious or cultural belief-system may feel that such traditions provide an adequate explanation for these phenomena. Persons who adopt a Christian or shamanic viewpoint, for example, may consider hostile and attacking voices which plague some mentally disturbed individuals to be the work of malevolent spirits. On the other hand, positive voice experiences which provide guidance, protection or companionship may be attributed to the presence of angels or protecting spirits.

It is important to note that a range of *psychological* explanations have been proposed to account for voices which appear to involve spirits. (Thomas Aquinas himself said that one should not resort to supernatural explanations for a phenomenon until all *natural* explanations have been exhausted.) Although these theories are often biased toward a narrowly materialistic view of the world there are nevertheless some which have been developed by highly sophisticated and spiritually aware researchers. For example, even though he described his patient's voices in terms of a realm of higher and lower order spirits, Wilson Van Dusen nevertheless speculated about the possible connection these experiences might have with the hearer's own psychological characteristics. In particular, he wondered whether viewing hallucinations as spirit presences on the one hand, or as dissociated ('split-off') aspects of the unconscious mind on the other, might not simply be two different ways of describing essentially the same thing:

> Are they really spirits or pieces of one's own unconscious? If the hallucinations came up with confirmably separate histories it would tend to confirm the spiritual hypothesis. We have already touched on the singular absence of a personal history and how this fits into the spirit model. In a way there are too many aspects of the matter that do not explain as well by the unconscious model as by the spiritual – consider for instance the gifts of the higher order spirits. The difference between the unconscious and spirit models grows darker when one considers that lower order spirits can only get in if they have tendencies like the person's own unconscious. Conversely I think higher order spirits only act in the direction of the individual's own higher, unconscious, unused potentialities. If this is so, it makes it difficult to separate them out as other than the person's own ... I would hope that further work might settle the matter for spirits or for a personal unconscious. But it might be that it is not either/or.[393]

It is widely agreed that voice experiences which appear to involve spirits can usually be adequately accounted for by psychological explanations which take into account the complex workings of the unconscious mind. For example, as was explained in Chapter Six, Jung felt that from a psychological perspective spirits could be understood in terms of projected autonomous complexes and archetypal images of the collective unconscious. Van Dusen himself noted that the higher order of voices 'looks most like Carl Jung's archetypes', whereas the lower order 'looks like Freud's id'.[394]

There may sometimes be more to it than this, however. As Van Dusen emphasised, it is not easy to account for the extraordinary wisdom demonstrated by voices of the higher order, nor for the resolutely anti-religious manner of the lower order. Undoubtedly this is a realm in which paradoxes and contradictions abound. A striking illustration of this fact was provided by Eileen Garrett, a medium who has had rigorous scientific testing. When she asked one of her spirit guides if she was seeing him or only something in her own brain she received a quite unexpected answer: 'both'![395] Interestingly, Jung himself appears to have had mixed feelings about this matter. Partly as a result of his own encounters with Philemon and other numinous figures from whom he received much important guidance and instruction, Jung remained open to the possibility that other explanations for these phenomena were sometimes warranted. Thus, whilst he remained sceptical in any particular case, he nevertheless stated:

> In actual practice one finds oneself again and again in the position of having to make do with the terminological crudities of science. I would like to draw a radical distinction between psychology as a science and psychology as a technique. In practice I have no compunction, if the case seems to be sufficiently certain, in speaking simply of spirits.[396]

It is clear that a great deal more research needs to be done by open-minded investigators before questions regarding the ultimate nature of spirits can be settled with any degree of certainty. In the meanwhile, the practical question of how best to respond to 'spirit' voices remains an issue of crucial importance.

The Importance of Discernment

While it is important to remain open-minded, anyone who hears voices which appear to be related to spirits or other supernatural agencies is strongly advised to exercise a great deal of caution in respect to them. Although such voices may sometimes be a source of profound comfort, inspiration and guidance, the possibility also exists that in some instances the hearer may be led astray, possibly even dangerously so. Furthermore, even if a voice experience has a genuinely benevolent spiritual origin it is always possible that the hearer may misunderstand or misinterpret its meaning. St Thomas Aquinas himself warned that even angels may sometimes be foes and tricksters of men.

Whether they are believed to come from within or without (e.g. whether it is a matter of malevolent spirits deliberately setting out to deceive or simply a person's own mind 'playing tricks' on them) great care should be taken in deciding how to respond to this kind of experience. The issue of discernment is especially relevant to people with a psychiatric disorder who hear voices which they believe have a supernatural origin (some voices may even explicitly claim such an identity).[397] Such beliefs are quite common among persons living with schizophrenia. Thus, for example, in a recent study of a group of twenty-six such people, *all* felt that their voices were omnipotent and omniscient and many attributed them to God, angels, the Devil, spirits of the dead or other non-human sources.[398] Because they are often experienced as being very powerful such voices have the potential to lead the hearer astray. People believing themselves to be acting in accordance with supernatural influences have occasionally carried out acts of violence against others or engaged in self-destructive behaviour, sometimes even leading to suicide. Furthermore, as Van Dusen frequently observed, a person's other-worldly experiences may provide the basis on which frankly delusional ideas eventually begin to develop:

> As the patient dealt more and more with the 'other world', even his vocabulary would change. Symbolic phrases that were learned there became a part of the patient's vocabulary. A whole set of ideas from the other world would be adopted, leaving the person technically delusional. It is hardly possible for an individual to experience a strange new world of experience some sixteen hours a day without it gradually colouring his whole view of reality.[399]

While it is possible that some of the voices heard by people with a psychiatric diagnosis may actually be helpful to them (e.g. higher order voices), there is also a risk that they could be harmed by others. This issue is further complicated by the fact that people who hear voices which they attribute to angels or devils often have great difficulty distinguishing between the two.[400] Van Dusen himself said that he could not always be sure which voices belonged to the higher order and which to the lower. He discovered, for example, that some voices which claimed to belong to the higher order were actually impostors from the lower order. Such fakery appears to be relatively common, as is borne out by the experience of a man living with schizophrenia who heard lower order voices which he called 'pursuers':

> As a matter of fact, certain pursuers, who are sadistic, have had a lot of 'fun' impersonating supernatural beings, and inducing and terrorising certain gullible persons into doing astonishing, terrible things. Certain pursuers have been able to get many persons to carry out their slightest wish, and these pursuers are evidently proud of their ability to do this. Being naturally, offensively domineering, they take delight in seeing what awful things they can get persons to do. Pursuers do not have to pretend to be supernatural. Different persons take it for granted; they consider pursuers must have the powers of the Holy Ghost.[401]

The Discernment of Spirits

Throughout history human beings have devised numerous means of protecting themselves from potentially harmful influences. Thus, for example, while spirits are accepted as an everyday reality in many non-Western cultures, strict guidelines nevertheless exist regarding who should attempt to contact them, and how and when this should be done. Furthermore, the wisdom of tribal elders, priests, and shamans is highly respected and relied upon to safeguard the participants in any socially-sanctioned ceremonies and healing rituals in which spirits are present.[402]

As was stated earlier the New Testament contains numerous references to the possible influence that spirits of various kinds might have on the lives of human beings. However, while they are accepted as a reality, it is acknowledged that their true nature and motives may not always be obvious. Thus, in traditional Christianity the importance of the so-called 'discernment of spirits' has always been very strongly emphasised since it involves the art of distinguishing genuinely benevolent spirits from impostors, and differentiating good influences from bad. The apostle John himself exhorted the faithful to 'test' all spirits:

> Beloved, do not believe every spirit, but test the spirits to see whether they are of God; for many false prophets have gone out into the world. (1 John 4: 1, RSV)

After spending many years studying the spirit-world the gifted Swedish spiritual teacher Emanuel Swedenborg* also gave stern warnings regarding the need for people to always be on guard against the ever-present potential for deception:

> When spirits begin to speak with man, he must beware lest he believe them in anything; for they say almost anything; things are fabricated by them, and they lie; for if they were permitted to relate what heaven is, and how things are in the heavens, they would tell so many lies, and indeed with solemn affirmation, that man would be astonished; wherefore, when spirits were speaking, I was not permitted to have faith in the things they related.[403]

Those who hear voices which seem to have a spiritual nature and origin are also urged to be wary of possible deception for there is always a risk of being led astray by negative or even frankly malevolent forces – some of which might disguise themselves so as to appear benevolent. St Teresa of Avila taught that spiritual locutions (voices) could be from God or the saints, the devil, or the hearer's own imagination, and that it was necessary to always exercise very great care in judging their true nature. The devil and his minions, she believed, could disguise themselves as angels, saints or other divine personages in order to deceive the unwary. In her famous treatise, *The Interior Castle*, St Teresa provided specific advice and guidance regarding the signs which help in discerning when there is deception and when there is not. The great Catholic mystic and spiritual teacher, St John of the Cross, also wrote at length on this subject in his book, *The Ascent of Mount Carmel*.

---

*Wilson Van Dusen was struck by the great similarity of his own findings regarding the 'higher' and 'lower' order hallucinations of his patients and the descriptions given by Swedenborg of the inhabitants of the spirit world.

Guidelines for Discernment

The guidelines below provide a simple and practical means of applying spiritual discernment to voice experiences which appear to have a supernatural origin.* It should be emphasised that in order for it to be complete and comprehensive discernment should always involve a consideration of both the *psychological* and the *spiritual* aspects of voice experiences.

Psychological Aspects of Discernment

Many voices which seem to have a supernatural origin can be explained in psychological terms. The saints of the Middle Ages pointed out that many apparently spiritual voice experiences actually originate in the imagination of the hearer. Over four centuries ago St John of the Cross expressed his concern about people who automatically assume their voices to be communications from God when in fact they are more often a product of the hearer's own fertile imagination:

> I greatly fear what is happening in these times of ours: If any soul whatever after a bit of meditation has ... one of these locutions [voices], it will immediately baptise all as coming from God and with such a supposition say, 'God told me,' 'God answered me.' Yet this is not so, but, as we pointed out, these persons themselves are more often the origin of their locution. Furthermore, their desire for such locutions and their attachment to them cause these persons to answer themselves and think that God is responding and speaking to them ... They think something extraordinary has occurred and that God has spoken, whereas in reality little more than nothing will have happened, or nothing at all, or even less than nothing ... some intellects are so lively and subtle that, while recollected in meditation, they reason naturally and easily about some concepts, and form locutions and propositions very vividly, and consequently

---

*As well as being applied to voices these guidelines might be helpful in establishing the spiritual veracity of a wide range of other experiences. For example, they could also be applied to beliefs, feelings or behaviours which either appear to have, or are claimed to have, a spiritual origin or nature.

think that these locutions are from God. But that notion is false, for an intellect, freed from the operation of the senses, has the capacity to do this and even more with its own natural light and without any other supernatural help. Such an occurrence is frequent. And many are deluded by it in thinking that theirs is the enjoyment of a high degree of prayer and communion with God; consequently they either write the words down themselves or have others do so. It comes about that the experience amounts to nothing, that no substantial virtue is derived from it, and that it serves for little more than inducing vainglory.[404]

The findings of modern research in depth psychology lend considerable support to the view that perceptions which involve 'spirits', 'demons' and other apparently supernatural entities can often be traced back to the unconscious psyche of the perceiver (see Chapter Six for an overview of relevant theories). For example, some voices which appear to be 'demons' may actually originate in the disowned and rejected aspects of the personality which Jung referred to as a person's 'shadow':

The psychological interpretation of the so-called 'demons' and 'ghosts' is that on some levels they are the embodied forms we give to our negative projections, those dark forces in ourselves which are too awful to admit into conscious-ness and which are then projected outward and turned against ourselves. In terms of Western psychology, these could be explained as ego-alien unconscious material and impulses that are projected as destructive forces that are perceived as an outer form which then possess us (audio-visual hallucinations, etc). Those are our own ghosts, so to speak . . . Ghosts are also the imprints of mental habits and thought patterns whose unconscious hold is so strong that they are constantly projected, unawares, onto the world . . . From the inner point of view, these 'demons' can also be explained as the negative archetypes of the collective unconscious, archetypes which overtake us from within.[405]

The psychological origin of apparently supernatural voices is sometimes revealed when their claims or identity are challenged.

For example, one of Van Dusen's female patients heard a voice which identified itself as Jesus Christ. He tested its claim to be able to read people's minds by asking the voice to tell him what he was thinking. It soon became obvious that it wasn't able to do what it said it could, which led the woman to begin doubting that it really was who it said it was. Eventually the voice left her. Two clinical psychologists have recently developed an approach which involves systematically disputing and challenging the identities of apparently omnipotent voices. They have used this approach to substantially reduce the distress experienced by a group of people living with schizophrenia who were initially convinced that their voices had supernatural power to control them.[406]

The fact that 'spirit' voices often speak in a highly symbolic manner often leads to doubt and uncertainty. People who take literally everything the voices say often remain ignorant of the hidden symbolic meaning of their communications. Following his own protracted struggle with the voices that he was once convinced were spirits, John Perceval eventually came to the realisation that their communications were meant to be understood metaphorically: 'The spirit speaks poetically but the man understands it literally'.[407] This realisation marked a significant turning-point in his struggle. Another man heard voices which claimed to be from Washington, DC, although they appeared to know nothing about this particular city. He eventually discovered that they were not referring to the city of Washington but rather to his own *inner* seat of government. Similarly, voices which say that something is 'poisonous' may be telling the hearer that it is bad for him or her and should therefore be avoided, not that it is physically poisonous.

Spiritual Aspects of Discernment

Over the centuries many spiritual traditions have amassed a wealth of experience relevant to the discernment of spirits. The following guidelines, which draw upon this accumulated wisdom, may be useful to anyone who hears voices which appear to have a supernatural origin.

(1) *Do not actively seek voice experiences*

Voice experiences of a spiritual kind are sometimes deliberately sought after by people hoping to gain some kind of benefit from them. However, spiritual traditions throughout the centuries have encouraged seekers to gratefully receive whatever God gives but not to deliberately seek out such experiences. Furthermore, since genuine spiritual experiences are ultimately a matter of grace they are a gift or blessing which cannot be produced at will. Many teachers warn that craving after spiritual experiences can amount to a kind of 'spiritual materialism' which will only increase the likelihood that the seeker will become subject to *false* experiences.

(2) *Try to ignore the voices*

Eastern spiritual traditions have long recognised that hallucination-like sensory experiences are a common occurrence during the practice of meditation, but such phenomena are usually considered to be potential distractions from the true spiritual path. Teachers of Zen Buddhist meditation, for example, instruct their students to ignore such phenomena which are thought of as 'makyo' (diabolical enticements). In the Christian tradition voices which are experienced as coming from *outside* the hearer (so-called 'corporeal locutions') are considered to be the most unreliable and therefore in need of especially cautious discernment, as St John of the Cross has explained:

> The more exterior and corporal they are, the less certain is their divine origin. God's communication is more commonly and appropriately given to the spirit, in which there is greater security and profit for the soul, than to the senses, where ordinarily there is extreme danger and room for deception ... He who esteems these [voices] is in serious error and extreme danger of being deceived. Or at least he will hinder his spiritual growth [because] these corporal perceptions bear no proportion to what is spiritual ... The more exterior these [voices], the less profitable they are to the interior and spiritual part of the soul ... they are a ready occasion for the breeding of error, presumption, and vanity.[408]

St Teresa advised that no attention should be paid to voices which originate in the hearer's own imagination. The safest attitude, according to St John, is to remain steadfast in resisting and rejecting *all* voices:

> The pure, cautious, simple, and humble soul should resist and reject revelations and other visions with as much effort and care as it would extremely dangerous temptations, for in order to reach the union of love there is no need of desiring them, but rather of rejecting them [for] to be perfect there is no need to desire to receive goods in a way that is supernatural and beyond one's capacity.[409]

Trying to ignore the voices minimises the risk of being misled. And, St John has assured, if the voices truly *are* from a higher spiritual source their beneficial effects will eventually become evident in the hearer's life anyway, despite the fact that every effort has been made to ignore them:

> Even though some may be from God, this rejection is no affront to Him, neither will one upon voluntarily dismissing them cease to receive the fruit God wishes to produce through these communications ... Since God grants these favours without the individual's own ability and effort, He causes the desired effect of these favours without this ability and effort, for this is an effect He produces passively in the spirit. The good effect, accordingly, does not depend upon wanting or not wanting the communication.[410]

(3) *Discuss voice experiences with others*

It is often very difficult for people to exercise reliable discernment on their own. For this reason most authorities insist that people should never accept apparently supernatural voices or act solely according to their own opinions about them without first seeking the advice and counsel of others. St John strongly emphasised this aspect of discernment:

> A person must not do what these words tell him, nor should he – whether they are from a good or bad spirit – pay any attention to them. Nevertheless, they should be manifested

to an experienced confessor or to a discreet and wise person who will give instructions and counsel and decide what is to be done ... It should be kept in mind that a person must never follow his own opinion, nor do or admit anything told to him through these locutions [voices], without ample advice and counsel from another. For in this matter of locutions strange and subtle deceits will occur – so much so that I believe a person who is unopposed to them cannot but be deceived in many.[411]

Discussing the complex issues raised by voice experiences with a trusted spiritual adviser such as a minister or priest, or with a mental health counsellor who has a sound understanding of spirituality, can be an invaluable aid in the effort to maintain a balanced perspective.

(4) *Study the personal effects of the voices*

All authorities agree that the only truly reliable way to determine whether or not an experience is from a benevolent spiritual source is to consider the effects it has on a person's life as a whole. Although genuine spiritual revelations which come in the form of voices may sometimes initially cause the hearer to experience fear and confusion, in time their effects always prove to be positive, beneficial and creative. On the other hand, some people have had voice experiences which initially caused feelings of elation and spiritual certainty only to find themselves being led into fear, doubt and despair by the same voices later on. The following are five widely accepted criteria relevant to this crucial aspect of discernment:

• *True spiritual experiences lead to an enhancement of calmness, peace, and love*
  The Bible lists the effects of God's spirit as these: love, joy, peace, patience, kindness, goodness, faithfulness, gentleness and self-control (Galatians 5:22–23, RSV). By contrast, experiences which result in agitation, fear and sadness, or which encourage isolation and separation from others, are likely to be of questionable origin.

• *Authentic spiritual experiences promote humility*
  The hearer should be wary of voices which lead to increased self-centredness or which cause them to feel special, important or proud, or which encourage the belief that they are better than

others for having these experiences. St Teresa especially emphasised this point:

> If the locutions [voices] contain words of favour and consolation from the Lord, let the soul look attentively to see if it thinks that because of them it is better than others. The more it hears words of favour the more humble it should be left; if it isn't, let it believe that the spirit is not from God. One thing very certain is that when the spirit is from God the soul esteems itself less, the greater the favour He granted, and it has more awareness of its sins and is more forgetful of its own gain, and its will and memory are employed more in seeking only the honour of God, nor does it think about its own profit, and it walks with greater fear lest its will deviate in anything, and with greater certitude that it never deserved any of these favours . . . [412]

- *Free will and critical reasoning should always be preserved*
  The hearer should be particularly wary of any voices which issue direct orders or demand blind obedience. Any influences which attempt to undermine a person's free will or diminish their ability to think for themselves are always suspect. As described earlier, the obsessing, possessing and compelling voices of the 'lower order' will often threaten or use actual force in an attempt to control or enslave the hearer.
- *Spiritual experiences generally conform to an authentic standard*
  One criterion for judging the authenticity of spiritual experiences involves determining the degree to which they conform to an accepted standard. Every spiritual tradition has a set of generally agreed upon principles and guidelines regarding the nature and workings of the spiritual life of human beings. Christians, for example, seek confirmation of the validity of their experiences in Biblical Scripture and in the life and works of Jesus Christ and exemplary personages such as the saints and other elevated souls.
- *Preoccupation with voices is generally an unhealthy sign*
  Truly spiritual voice experiences tend to occur only once or at most occasionally or intermittently (although there can be exceptions to this general rule). Voices which persist over longer periods of time may therefore be questionable. Furthermore, while voice experiences may foster and enhance a person's interest in spiritual practices and religious observances, becoming

preoccupied or obsessed with these matters is usually an undesirable sign.

(5) *Do not act on voice experiences*

A final safeguard against possible error and deception involves the hearer refusing to comply with any suggestions or commands the voices might make. St Teresa was adamant that by taking this course the beneficial effects of true spiritual experiences would still occur, but that any potential dangers would be minimised. She felt that even if a voice came from the devil himself the hearer would be protected from deception as long as they recognised the absence of the favourable signs listed above, remained humble, and steadfastly refused to act:

> In my opinion the devil will say the words very clearly so that there will be certitude about their meaning, as is so with those coming from the Spirit of truth. But he will not be able to counterfeit the effects that were mentioned [under point number (4) above] or leave this peace and light in the soul; on the contrary he leaves restlessness and disturbance. But he can do little or no harm if the soul is humble and does what I have mentioned, that is, doesn't make a move to do a thing of what it hears.[413]

St John of the Cross pointed out that even if a particular voice experience had a diabolical origin its effects would not be lasting as long as it was resisted by the hearer:

> Yet diabolical communications are not as efficacious in doing harm as God's communications are in doing good. For the diabolical communications can only arouse the first movements without being able to move the will any further if it is unwilling to be moved. The unrest caused by them will not last long, unless the individual's lack of courage and circumspection occasion its endurance.[414]

In the final analysis it may be impossible to reach any absolute degree of certainty regarding the identity and source of many apparently spiritual voices. In light of this, the guidelines listed above can provide a sound and well-tested basis for a pragmatic approach to evaluating the nature and effects of such experiences, while at the same time helping to safeguard the hearer and others from possible harm.

Conclusion

With the resurgence of interest in spirituality that is evident throughout the Western world many people now readily accept the possibility of being able to communicate with non-physical entities such as spirit guides and various other 'messengers' from beyond the boundaries of the material world. As witness to this, the December 27, 1993 edition of *Time* magazine devoted its cover story to the phenomenon of angels, reporting that two out of every three people in the USA believe in their existence, and one person in three claims to have felt an angelic presence in their life at some time. In recent years angels have been the subject of many books (including some best-sellers), numerous magazine articles, and a number of television programmes. Although they have generally been ignored by the mainstream scientific, theological and psychological establishments a number of reputable scholars have begun discussing and writing about them.[415]

Those who are inclined to be sceptical may find it rather tempting to dismiss the whole matter of spirits (and related phenomena, such as trance-channelling) as evidence of the excesses of shallow, pseudo-religious 'New Age' thinking – if it is not simply a question of charlatanism or self-delusion. Much of what passes for New Age wisdom *is* undoubtedly of questionable spiritual value. Indeed, in view of the very real dangers of spiritual pride and deception, the need for cautious discernment is possibly greater now than it has ever been. Some popular contemporary practitioners of channelling – such as those who 'either write the words down themselves or have others do so' – would undoubtedly find the counsel of St John of Cross rather challenging! With the prescience that is borne of true spiritual maturity he warned more than four hundred years ago that 'in this matter of locutions strange and subtle deceits will occur'.

Those who do not dismiss outright all experiences that are claimed to be connected with spirits may choose to describe them as intrapsychic phenomena. As explained above, dissociation and various other psychological mechanisms can indeed be invoked in order to account for many supposedly supernatural experiences. In spite of these endeavours (which have sometimes been known to distort the facts in an attempt to fit a cherished theory) it is clear that such explanations cannot yet adequately account for many aspects of the kinds of experience described in this chapter. Consequently, until further research has been done and a great deal more evidence accumulated, the only intellectually honest attitude is one which leaves open the possibility that there may be influential realms beyond the physical – as traditional cultures readily accept and as Christianity and other spiritual traditions have long maintained. Along with many ordinary people a growing number of scientists and other scholars now accept this possibility.

One of the most eloquent of those who have argued in favour of remaining open-minded about these issues was Daniel Paul Schreber, a nineteenth century German supreme court judge whose autobiographical account of an experience of psychosis is one of the most influential of such first-person accounts ever written.[416] When Schreber's *Memoirs Of My Nervous Illness* first appeared in 1903 it was discussed by many of the important pioneers of psychiatry and analysed by Sigmund Freud, who subsequently based a number of his theories upon its contents. While in the throes of a protracted and extremely florid psychosis Schreber became convinced that he was a 'seer of spirits': a person who sees and is in communication with spirits or departed souls. When he recovered Schreber remained adamant that, while many of his experiences were undoubtedly hallucinatory, there may have been rather more to it than this. He pleaded for both an open-minded and genuinely scientific approach to these matters rather than the usual hasty dismissal of them:

> The legends and poetry of all peoples literally swarm with the activities of ghosts, elves, goblins, etc., and it seems to me nonsensical to assume that in all of them one is dealing simply with deliberate inventions of human imagination without any foundation in real fact ... I do not dispute that in many of these cases one may only be dealing with mere hallucinations [but] in my opinion science would go very wrong to designate as 'hallucinations' all such phenomena that lack objective reality, and to throw them into the lumber room of things that do not exist ... Therefore one ought to beware of unscientific generalisation and rash

condemnation in such matters . . . If psychiatry is not flatly
to deny everything supernatural and thus tumble with both
feet into the camp of naked materialism, it will have to
recognise the possibility that occasionally the phenomena
under discussion may be connected with real happenings,
which simply cannot be brushed aside with the catchword
'hallucinations'.[417]

Echoing Schreber's plea it might be said that no contemporary
approach to hearing voices can claim to be complete unless it
includes a sincere attempt to understand the phenomenon of 'spirits'
since these experiences – whatever they are – appear to be rooted
in the deepest levels of the human mind and soul.

Chapter Eight

COPING WITH DISTURBING VOICES

Half the power of a symptom is relieved by understanding its
cause and how to avoid having it become worse . . . What
power and joy it was to feel relief and to have something
with which to attack these terrible monsters of my soul.
— Marcia Lovejoy[418]

Hearing voices is a frightening and disturbing experience for some people and all they want is for it to stop and for the voices to go away and leave them alone. Fear and distress provoked by voices may be related to the specific contents of what they say (e.g. harsh criticism, insults, threats), the hostile, insulting or derisive manner in which they speak, or to both their content and their manner of speaking. In addition, many people are afraid that the actual fact of hearing voices must mean that they are no longer the person they were and that they are, instead, certifiably 'crazy' or 'insane'. Considerable fear can accompany voice experiences even if the voices themselves are friendly and say mainly positive things. For example, people who have genuinely spiritual voices sometimes feel quite fearful initially and some even try to actively resist the experience.

One of the main causes of distress for many people relates to their fear of losing control. In extreme cases the hearer may feel that they have become a passive victim at the mercy of powerful external forces which are completely beyond comprehension. What some people find particularly distressing is the feeling that someone or something else has gained control over their mind and is able to manipulate their thoughts and feelings at will. Some people feel especially concerned about the fact that their innermost personal space and privacy has been intruded upon by an uninvited 'other', often one they can neither see nor speak back to. Rachel Corday has graphically described the peculiarly invasive quality of the kind

195

of voices which many people experience at times during the emotional turmoil of acute psychosis:

> In psychosis, these voices come uninvited. We do not sit and meditate and welcome entities to use us. We are invaded, imposed upon as if a thief has broken into our home, pushed us aside, eaten our food, broken our belongings, and is sleeping in our bed.[419]

Despite the fact that they often have the potential to cause fear and distress not everyone necessarily wants their voice experiences to stop completely. Some people feel that even though the voices are sometimes nasty to them they nevertheless have some positive aspects. For example, some people enjoy having their voices pay attention to them, while others say that hearing voices makes them feel special or important. As well as being someone to talk things over with the voices may challenge the hearer to do things that would be good for them. Some voices even tell jokes! Many people experience their voices as sources of valued companionship or guidance, perhaps even of inspiration. Because hearing voices can involve such a mixture of different experiences it frequently has both positive and negative aspects. This is especially likely to be the case for people who have been hearing voices for some time and who have adjusted to their presence and found ways to cope with them.

Many people who are disturbed by voices discover through personal experience that there are things they can do to decrease their distress and increase their sense of control. Some learn to stop the voices altogether while others eventually develop an ability to live more comfortably with them. In every case a process of trial-and-error is involved since each person must discover for him or herself what works best and suits their own particular needs and circumstances. It is especially important to remember that, since hearing voices is an experience which occurs within the total context of the hearer's life, it can only be properly understood and effectively dealt with by adopting an *holistic approach* in which every aspect of the hearer's life and being – body, mind and soul – is taken into account.

In this chapter the basic principles relevant to coping successfully with disturbing voices are described under the following three main headings:

(1) Reducing the fear of voices
(2) Preventing voices from occurring
(3) Learning to control the voices

(1) *REDUCING THE FEAR OF VOICES*

Because many people in Western societies still consider it to be an indication of 'madness' the experience of hearing voices is often feared and heavily stigmatised. By contrast, fear and stigma are often much lower (or even completely absent) in many non-Western societies where voices and other unusual kinds of experience are accepted and given supernatural or other non-stigmatising and culturally valued explanations.[420] In fact, experiences which Westerners generally tend to think of as 'hallucinations' may be highly valued or even revered in some parts of the world. In many societies voices and visions are actively sought after and various techniques (e.g. prolonged fasting, sleep deprivation, solitude, spiritual practices) may be used in an attempt to deliberately induce them. An anecdote reported by Dr Richard Warner, a psychiatrist and anthropologist who has studied attitudes to psychosis in Third World societies, clearly illustrates the fact that far more tolerant social attitudes toward voice experiences exist in many non-Western cultures:

> In many cases where a supernatural explanation for psychotic features is used, the label 'crazy' or 'insane' may never be applied. I once remarked to a Sioux mental health worker from the Pine Ridge Reservation in South Dakota that most Americans who heard voices would be diagnosed as psychotic. Her response was simple: 'That's terrible.'[421]

Despite the popular association of voices with 'madness' in Western societies the fact that a person hears voices does *not* in itself necessarily indicate that they are psychotic or in any way 'mentally ill'. Psychiatrists consider psychosis to be a complex mental state which always involves a disturbance of *many* aspects of a person's behaviour, including their thinking processes and emotions. Furthermore, psychotic disorders are specifically characterised by a gross impairment of the affected person's contact with reality and a significant deterioration in their level of personal, social, and occupational functioning. Consequently, nobody could ever legitimately be considered psychotic solely on the basis of their experience of hearing voices.

It is instructive to discover just how common voice-hearing experiences actually are. As was extensively documented in the first part of this book, many well-adjusted, highly successful and creative individuals have heard voices. Such experiences have undoubtedly played a significant role in the development of the world's major religious movements as well as in many of the minor ones. Apart from this, many otherwise quite ordinary individuals have had experiences involving voices. For example, during bereavement it is quite common for people to see, hear or even speak with the recently deceased person. Over 70% of the 'normal' college students interviewed for the study described in Chapter One said that they had occasionally heard voices while fully awake. If it is assumed that voice experiences occur with a similar frequency in the general population it would seem reasonable to conclude that it is actually rather unusual for a human being *not* to have heard a voice at least once in their life! (As a matter of fact it is likely that the true frequency of voice experiences is even higher than this research has suggested since fear and stigma probably causes some people to deny ever having had them.) The views expressed in an article published in the *American Journal of Psychiatry* in 1983 neatly summarise the current situation:

> Most persons who have hallucinations are not in any way mentally ill. Many members of the general population seem to have had one or several memorable hallucinatory experiences ... Most persons who have unusual sensory experiences tell few people, or no one about them. They rarely know that many other people have had similar experiences and have also remained silent for fear of being considered abnormal ... They have heard that hallucinations are symptoms of insanity, and they have no way of knowing that such experiences are not necessarily indicators of mental illness, either present or to come.[422]

Meeting and sharing experiences with other people who hear voices or who simply have an open-minded interest in them can be an important source of comfort and support and undoubtedly helps to reduce feelings of fear and isolation. Just knowing that many others have had similar experiences can itself be very reassuring. Reading and learning about voices also helps to diminish ignorance and misunderstanding and is therefore invaluable both to people who hear voices and to those involved in providing support.

Note: The 'Recommended Reading' section at the end of this book contains a list of books and articles suitable for the general reader. Details of support groups and other relevant resources are listed in the Appendix.

(2) PREVENTING VOICES FROM OCCURRING

When voices first start they often seem to come and go at random which may leave the hearer feeling that they have absolutely no control over when, where and how often they occur. However, in time many people gradually discover that the voices are *not* actually a totally random occurrence and that they tend to hear them only when they are in specific situations or in a particular mood or frame of mind. Once a person has learnt to identify the circumstances which seem to 'trigger' the onset of their voices it may then become possible to selectively avoid these particular kinds of situations and thereby prevent the voices from beginning in the first place.

The specific 'triggers' which cause a person's voices to begin tend to be very individual so that a situation which stimulates the onset of one person's voices may not necessarily have the same effect on another. Very often it is how a particular situation makes a person *feel* that determines how they will respond to it – including whether or not it causes their voices to start. While there are very many possible 'triggers' for voices the five listed below appear to be particularly common. Sometimes the voices may be triggered by a combination of different factors acting together (such as a high level of stress *and* a low level of auditory stimulation).

(a) Stress and Emotional Arousal

Stress of various kinds (e.g. crowds of people, family conflict, arguments, excessive pressure to perform, loneliness, anger, frustration) often seems to trigger voices or causes them to become even more intense if they are already present.[423] When stressed some people may (unconsciously) begin to hyperventilate which in itself can trigger the onset of voices in certain individuals.[424] More specifically, many people seem most likely to hear voices when they are feeling troubled by some particular emotional conflict such as guilt or anger. For example, a person who feels he has failed at something may subsequently be attacked and belittled by critical voices which add to the intensity of his sense of inadequacy. Some people discover that their voices tend to become worse when they have significant personal issues which they are not dealing with. Being under pressure to make difficult decisions may also cause high levels of stress, and at such times some people may begin to hear voices which they feel help or guide them in deciding what to do. Maryanne Handel has described how her voices began whenever she became highly stressed:

> I had gotten into a situation of stress and conflict in the place I was living with a couple of other people, and I was under a lot of stress and I had a lot of anger. I was furious and I was getting very overwrought. I couldn't switch off all these distracting thoughts which were causing me a lot of stress, and I started to sleep very badly and then I started hearing the voices again.[425]

By selectively avoiding excessively stressful situations and learning to use effective stress management techniques many people are able to reduce both the frequency and the intensity of voices which are triggered by stress. Some people teach themselves to use pre-learned relaxation techniques *as soon as they start hearing voices* so that they can prevent themselves from getting caught in the 'vicious circle' of escalating anxiety which may begin when the voices start up. If a person can remain calm even though they are hearing disturbing voices the voices may eventually begin to diminish or even disappear completely.

(b) Expectation

People often seem to only hear voices when they are in a particular mood or frame of mind. For example, John Perceval discovered that he only heard voices when he allowed himself to enter into an 'absent' state of mind:

> I found, moreover, if I threw myself back into the same state of absence of mind, that the voice returned, and I subsequently observed that the style of address would

appear to change according to the mood of mind I was in; still later, while I was continuing these observations, I found that although these voices usually come to me without thought on my part, I had sometimes a power, to a certain extent, to choose what I would hear.[426]

Some people learn that they hear voices talking about them only when they are actually *expecting* to hear them. For instance, one woman could be at work all day without hearing any voices but she expected to hear her neighbours talking about her and when she returned home and listened for them she did hear them. A psychiatrist, Dr Silvano Arieti, coined the term 'listening attitude' to describe the particular expectant mood that often seems to precede the onset of voices:

Hallucinatory voices occur only in particular situations, that is, *when the patient expects to hear them* . . . In other words, he puts himself in what I have called *the listening attitude* . . . he puts himself into this attitude when he is in a particular situation or in a particular mood, for instance, a mood in which he perceives hostility almost in the air. He feels that everybody has a disparaging attitude toward him. Then he finds corroboration for this attitude of others; he hears them making unpleasant remarks about him.[427]

By paying close attention to the frame of mind they are in immediately before their voices begin some people are eventually able to see that there is a close connection between their mood and the onset of voices. Some therapists attempt to help people become aware of how the intensity of their voices increases when they are feeling stressed and *expect* that their voices will become audible. A person who recognises that certain moods or patterns of thinking (such as negative 'self talk') precede the onset of their voices may eventually be able to prevent the voices from occurring by learning how to control or avoid these particular mental states. John Perceval eventually learnt to avoid the 'absent' state of mind that coincided with the onset of his voices:

He found that [his] openness to his sensory environment was chronically being interrupted and covered over by a mechanism that felt like a 'film', or a 'fog', insidiously descending over his mind and clouding his awareness.

Inevitably, he found himself projecting images onto this film, images that became animated, thus cutting him off from external sensory awareness. He finally solved this riddle by practicing at becoming quick enough to recognise the subtle sensation of the film as it first came to him, and then cutting through it. Thus, the sensation of the film itself became his moment of 'recollection', the reminder to wake himself up.[428]

As a person comes to recognise that the occurrence of voices is connected with their mood or frame of mind they will no longer feel like a totally passive victim at the mercy of invisible forces. On the contrary, they will increasingly understand that their mental and emotional states play a key role in determining what they experience.

(c) Low Levels of Auditory Stimulation

People are most likely to hear voices during periods of prolonged social isolation and inactivity. This is actually not particularly surprising since it is known that *many* people will eventually begin to hallucinate if they are exposed to conditions of extreme isolation and sensory under-stimulation such as occur during sensory deprivation experiments. As described in Chapter One astronauts, polar explorers, light-house keepers, and solitary sailors have all experienced hallucinations after spending prolonged periods of time alone. Researchers have found that people are especially likely to hear voices if they are exposed to continuous, unvarying sound which contains little or no information and which does not engage their attention (this kind of sound is sometimes referred to as 'white noise').[429]

Voices are especially common when a stressed or emotionally aroused person is exposed to a constant, low level of unpatterned sound (e.g. the low rumble of background traffic, the drone of machinery, or the hum of domestic appliances such as air-conditioners or electric hair-driers). For practical purposes this means that some people may be able to prevent or eliminate their voices by increasing the amount of auditory stimulation they receive (e.g. deliberately listening to sounds which contain information and command attention, engaging in conversation with others, or getting involved in some kind of activity). *Some practical applications of these ideas are discussed in detail under the heading 'Auditory Stimulation' later in this chapter.*

(d) Physical Health Problems

Voice experiences can occur as a result of disturbances of physiological functioning such as those associated with a variety of medical disorders and conditions. People who are troubled by disturbing voices sometimes find that changes in their physical health can lead to a temporary increase in voice frequency or intensity. For example, some women notice that they have more problems with their voices during the premenstrual phase of their menstrual cycle. Even relatively minor physical illnesses can sometimes have this effect, as Marcia Lovejoy discovered:

> The psychiatrist who saw me in 1972 ... has gone over my hospital records and found that 40 percent of the time I came in with a previously undiagnosed physical ailment such as pneumonia, cystitis, or anaemia. When these conditions cleared up so did my psychiatric problems. Based on this finding, he later asked me to take my temperature the next time I hallucinated. At first I thought he was kidding, but I followed his orders and did find a correlation between raised temperature and psychotic symptoms. Taking my temperature became an important tool in my life ... which helped me feel less out of control.[430]

The possible effect that a person's diet and lifestyle might have on their voices is presently unknown. However, some people living with schizophrenia have found that certain foods seem to cause their symptoms to worsen while other foods or dietary supplements (such as vitamins) may have a beneficial effect. Paying careful attention to general health, fitness, and diet undoubtedly helps some people to minimise problems with voices. For example, Norma MacDonald discovered how important it is to get adequate rest and maintain a proper diet:

> I *must* have three square meals, my necessary nutrients, and at least eight hours sleep nightly ... I know that by going

without food for a day or two or by missing sleep two or three nights in a row I could (and do) lapse into a state where dreams worry my mind at night, fatigue sets in, voices begin to pester me, and suspicions of the motives of even my best friends rises up . . . [431]

(e) Alcohol and Drug Use

Many drugs are known to cause people to experience hallucinations. Psychedelic drugs such as LSD ('acid'), mescaline ('peyote'), and psylocibin ('magic mushrooms') are also known as 'hallucinogens' since they can induce hallucinatory experiences of one kind or another in most people who take them. Marijuana ('dope', 'grass', 'hash', 'pot') and stimulant drugs such as amphetamines ('speed') can also cause hallucinations. Under certain circumstances all of these drugs can induce a psychotic state (i.e. a 'drug-induced psychosis') in which hallucinations occur, though they usually disappear as the effects of the drug wear off. People withdrawing from heavy alcohol abuse sometimes experience hallucinations while in delirium tremens ('DTs'). This state usually only lasts for a few days, although occasionally a person who has recovered from the symptoms of alcohol withdrawal and is no longer drinking will continue to hear voices (this is referred to as 'alcoholic hallucinosis').

Although it is not known at present what specific effect commonly used social drugs such as nicotine (in tobacco), caffeine (in coffee, tea, chocolate, and some cola drinks), and alcohol might have on voices it is possible that *excessive* use of these substances could be problematic. Many people with a psychiatric diagnosis seem to be especially sensitive to the effects of both social and illicit drugs. Furthermore, it is now known that nicotine tends to counteract the effects of the neuroleptic ('anti-psychotic') drugs which some people take to help control voices.[432]

The following questions may be useful in helping people to identify some of the inner and outer factors that may influence the timing, duration, content and other specific qualities of their voices:

• Do your voices tend to occur at any particular times or in any specific situations?

- Are there certain times when they are louder or more aggressive and others when they are quieter or more friendly?
- Is voice frequency and content affected by your mood or frame of mind?
- Is what the voices say related in some way to how you are feeling about yourself at the time you hear them?
- Are the voices affected by your diet, alcohol intake, consumption of caffeine, nicotine, or other drugs?
- Are they affected by your state of general health? (e.g. diet, fever, menstruation)
- Are there any other factors you can identify which seem to affect the voices for better or worse?

In attempting to answer these questions it can be helpful to have a trusted friend or counsellor to discuss them with. A diary can be used as an aid to help identify any patterns or reactions that might not be immediately obvious.

(3) *LEARNING TO CONTROL THE VOICES*

A significant source of distress for many people results from the feeling that they have little control over the voices. Hostile, attacking and intrusive voices are especially likely to provoke fear and anxiety. However, in time most people who hear disturbing voices are able to learn some ways to handle them more effectively so that their sense of control gradually becomes stronger.

On a *social level* a degree of control can be gained as a person learns to suppress what may be their natural and spontaneous response to these experiences. For example, many people learn that it is usually better not to talk back to voices in public. A person's actions always speak louder than their voices! Thus, by learning to maintain control over their outwardly observable behaviour, the hearer can ensure that no one else ever knows about their inner (voice) experiences unless they choose to talk about them. Another control measure involves a voice hearer using common sense to guide their decisions about when and with whom they can safely discuss their experiences. One man gave the following simple advice regarding such disclosure:

I have plenty of friends and many of them know about me and help me in various ways. However, not all of them want to hear about my experiences, so that in one's social life perhaps it is advisable to keep quiet about these, especially where sympathy is lacking.[433]

While this kind of social control can be extremely important many people who hear voices also find great relief in being able to share their experiences openly with others who are tolerant, accepting and understanding. Sharing in this way can result in a significant improvement in social and emotional problems such as isolation and anxiety.

On a more *personal level* the hearer's distress can often be significantly reduced if they are able to gain some degree of direct control of the voices and there are at least two ways in which this is often possible. Firstly, some people learn that they can prevent their voices from beginning in the first place by avoiding the kinds of situations that tend to 'trigger' them (see the discussion above). Secondly, there are a wide range of quite simple techniques which many people have found to be effective in stopping their voices or at least reducing their frequency and intensity. By using one or both of these approaches many people are able to significantly reduce their distress and enhance their sense of control. This in itself may actually help to reduce the frequency or the intensity of the voices since anxiety and stress often tend to make them worse.

There are a very wide range of strategies and techniques which can be useful for gaining control over voices. Some of the methods described below were actually discovered by people who were troubled by voices and who experimented with different ways of trying to make them stop. Others were devised by therapists and researchers.[434] Anyone wishing to control or eliminate disturbing voices may find some of these methods effective. Choosing a particular technique to use may be partly determined by convenience. For example, some may be more suitable for use in private (e.g. reading aloud) while others can be used in public (e.g. stereo headphones). Because of the highly individual nature of voice experiences the only sure way to discover if any of these techniques will work is to actually try it out. A reasonable amount of time and effort should be devoted to learning and practising the techniques since it can sometimes take a while to achieve the desired results.

Using a combination of different techniques rather than just a single one will often prove to be most effective.

Techniques that may help a person to control or stop their voices include the following:

1 Distraction	12 Reasoning with the Voices
2 Vocal Activity	13 Challenging the Voices
3 Relaxation	14 First Person Singular Therapy
4 Interpersonal Contact	15 Selective Listening
5 Physical Stimulation	16 Cultivating Self-Esteem
6 Auditory Stimulation	17 Maintaining Positive Attitudes
7 Ignoring the Voices	and Expectations
8 Dismissing the Voices	18 Restricting or Avoiding
9 Thought Stopping	Non-Prescription Drugs
10 Aversion Therapy	19 Psychotropic Medications
11 Self-Monitoring	20 Miscellaneous Strategies

1 *Distraction*

Many people find that deliberately shifting attention away from the voices and onto something outside of themselves helps to alleviate their distress.[435] Some people may even be able to forget about their voices completely if they keep busy or get involved in activities of various kinds. A very wide range of activities may be effective in distracting attention away from voices: socialising with other people, listening to music, watching television, reading, writing, work, hobbies or handicrafts, housework, gardening, playing sports, and so on. A change of environment can also help to shift attention onto other things (e.g. going for a walk or drive, visiting people, shopping, and so on). Activities and tasks that require full attention are likely to be most effective since they require a person to put their mind onto something other than the voices. It is naturally much easier for people to fully engage their attention in an activity if it involves doing something they find interesting or personally rewarding.

In time some people may learn to catch themselves when they are in the specific 'listening attitude' (described earlier) which often seems to precede the onset of voices. At such times if they consciously and deliberately start to do something which engages their attention (e.g. starting up a conversation with someone), they may be able to 'snap' themselves out of this frame of mind and thus prevent voices from beginning. Sometimes, *other* people (such as friends or family members) who have learnt to recognise the tell-tale signs of the 'listening attitude' may be able to distract the person's attention before their voices begin.

2 *Vocal Activity*

It has been observed that some people whisper quietly to themselves while they are hearing voices (the 'Subvocal Speech' theory of voices was discussed in Chapter Six). Although it is not known exactly what connection there may be between this kind of subvocal whispering and voices, some people are able to make their voices stop by deliberately engaging in a vocal activity which prevents them from using their vocal chords for whispering.[436] There are several quite simple ways to do this:

• Speaking to someone
• Humming or singing quietly to oneself
• Counting or repeating a mantra under the breath
• Reading aloud
• Yawning, gargling or simply holding one's mouth open wide

These methods can be very effective in stopping voices while they are actually being used and some people may find that they also have a long-term effect (e.g. the voices stop and don't come back again).

3 *Relaxation*

As well as helping to diminish the hearer's distress inducing a state of deep relaxation can have the effect of reducing the frequency of disturbing voices or possibly even cause them to stop. A wide variety of methods may be effective for these purposes including progressive muscular relaxation and stress-reducing forms of meditation such as Transcendental Meditation (TM). Some people discover for themselves through a process of trial-and-error how to use relaxation to control their voices. For example, Maryanne

Handel learnt to use a particular breathing technique which she developed herself:

> I found that I could sort of breathe it out. If I relaxed and just breathed like so [gently inhaling and exhaling] I'd be able to breathe it away, and then I relaxed again and the voice would fade and retreat.[437]

It is often easiest for a person to learn and practise relaxation techniques when they are *not* hearing any voices. Then, once they have become confident in their ability to induce a state of relaxation, they will have a useful 'tool' which they can use if and when the voices begin. Some people who only hear voices when they are tense or anxious may even be able to learn to relax sufficiently to prevent the voices from occurring in the first place. People whose voices become worse when they are overstimulated by stress or emotional pressure may find it helpful to use *temporary* social withdrawal in order to give themselves some necessary 'time out'. For example, one woman found that isolating herself for a short time in her bathroom gave her a chance to calm down, relax and regain self-control. One man has described how he learnt to use a self-taught technique he termed 'systematic de-conditioning' to help him master his disturbing hallucinatory voices:

> When applying systematic de-conditioning to my halluci-nations, all I did was to sit down, relax completely (as I had been taught previously in hospital), and then run through in my mind all the hallucinations that were worrying me, in increasing order of terror. As soon as I found myself tightening up I would stop, re-relax, and go back to the beginning, starting again with the least frightening hallucination. Once I had mastered hallucinat-ions in this way I was able to use the system for coming to terms with many things that had up to then worried me in real life . . . [438]

The technique this man called 'systematic de-conditioning' is very similar to systematic de-sensitisation, a standard technique used by many clinical psychologists. It basically involves a person learning to remain relaxed while they are systematically exposed to anxiety-provoking situations or stimuli of gradually increasing intensity.

4 Interpersonal Contact

Many people who hear voices find that it can help to make contact with others. For example, those whose voices become worse when they are alone and isolated may find that interacting with others brings some relief. Simply being with a friend or a trusted companion -- without necessarily talking or doing anything in particular – may be very comforting at times. As well as the fact that being with others can help to distract a person's attention away from themselves the very act of speaking sometimes has the specific effect of making voices stop.[439] (This may be related to the fact that speaking requires a person to utilise their vocal chords – see 'Vocal Activity' above.) Conversation does not necessarily have to involve talking about voices – everyday subjects of interest can be equally effective. When direct personal contact with others is not possible (or is not desired) telephoning, or even writing to them, may suffice. The advent of computer networking now makes it possible to have safe interactive contact with a very wide range of people.

5 Physical Stimulation

Some people may find that changing their level of physical arousal – either increasing or decreasing it – can help to reduce or eliminate voices. Voices which occur when a person is experiencing a high level of arousal (e.g. excessive stress, emotional over-stimulation) can sometimes be reduced by engaging in calming activities such as relaxation exercises, sleep, or listening to soothing music. Some people have found that physical immobility, achieved by sitting or lying quietly, is helpful. There have even been reports of people whose voices ceased altogether when they adopted certain physical postures. When voices are associated with a *low* level of arousal stimulating physical exercise such as walking or jogging can help. Some people find that vigorous physical exercise such as running, swimming, playing sports, or aerobics is very effective.[440]

6 Auditory Stimulation

Some people may be able to control their voices by either increasing or decreasing the amount of auditory stimulation they receive. The following are two simple and practical ways of doing this:

(a) Earplugs:

In a recent experimental study over 50% of the people who wore an earplug (the kind that people sometimes wear at loud rock concerts or while swimming) whenever they heard voices over a period of one week reported experiencing some benefit and in several cases the voices disappeared completely for several months afterwards.[441] It should be noted that using an earplug often seems to have a rather variable effect. For instance, it may be more effective in one ear than in the other, or the voices may stop *after* but not while the person is wearing it.[442] For these reasons anyone who uses an earplug should experiment with it in each ear and insert it for different periods of time in order to discover what works best for them. For example, the earplug could initially be worn in the left ear to see what effect it has. If there has been no change in the voices after a while it should be switched to the right ear. A little patience is required as this technique can take some time to work. The advantage of using earplugs (rather than headphones, as described below) is that they are inconspicuous and do not interfere with a person's ability to perform other activities.

(b) Headphones:

Many people who are troubled by voices find that listening to music, radio, or TV programmes can provide temporary relief. In general it has been found that anything which produces an increase in external auditory stimulation (i.e. sound) may help to reduce the intensity of voices. Listening to music through headphones connected to a portable radio-cassette player (such as a 'Walkman') can often be an effective way to control voices.[443] Some people listen to loud, stimulating music in an attempt to 'drown out' their voices but researchers have found that the loudness of the sound does not seem to be the most important factor. Headphones usually work best when what is listened to is interesting and meaningful and fully engages the listener's attention. If the music or talk is not very interesting it is less likely to help control the voices.[444] Anyone interested in trying this method should experiment with different kinds of music or radio programmes (e.g. talk-back, sports broadcasts) in order to discover what is most effective. The disadvantage of headphones is that they may sometimes restrict social interaction and it may not always be possible to use them in any situation when they are needed. On the positive side, radio-cassette players are relatively cheap, portable, socially acceptable, fully under the control of the user, do not disturb anyone else – and cause no side-effects!

An illustration of the effectiveness of headphones can be found in the experiences of a man who continued to be troubled by a voice despite taking prescribed neuroleptic medication. He bought a portable cassette player and made a tape to play whenever he heard the voice. At first he used a tape of himself shouting back at the voice but it did not help. He then decided to record and play pleasant memories of his family, work and holidays. He listened to this tape whenever he heard the voice and found that, within a few minutes of putting it on, the voice disappeared. After fifteen months of using this tape he still found it to be the only truly effective way to make the voice stop.[445]

7 *Ignoring the Voices*

Some people are able to control troubling voices by deliberately excluding them from awareness. The following comments were made by people describing how they handled their voices: 'I ignore them'; 'Get them off my mind'; 'Avoid it, like static on a radio – tune out'; 'Think of sending the voice away and it goes away'; 'I push the voices aside'.[446] Maryanne Handel was initially angry at the voices and visions which bothered her, but she eventually discovered that she could stop them:

> One day I got angry with them for sending all these thoughts and images which I didn't want. So I said angrily, 'I don't have to see anything I don't want to see!', just like that. Meaning it was my right, it was just outrageous. I just said 'I don't have to see anything I don't want to see', very angry. And then something sort of twigged and I thought, 'Well, even if somebody is sending me these images, I bet I can do something to shut them out if I want to. I bet I don't have to put up with this. If I want to I can do something with my mind to shut it out.' So I kept saying that, I kept saying, 'I don't have to see anything I don't want to see', over

and over again. And when I did that it worked, it would fade, it would go away.[447]

Some people try to block out all thoughts and 'empty' their minds completely but this is difficult to do. Ignoring voices often works best if at the same time the hearer attempts to occupy their mind with pleasant or positive thoughts and keeps busy with some interesting activity. It is possible for a person to improve their ability to ignore voices if they practise deliberately ignoring distracting sounds. For example, a person could practise listening to a friend or helper who speaks to them while a TV or radio is on in the background. After a while of doing this it will gradually become easier to focus on the conversation and ignore the distracting sounds of the TV or radio. The skills which a person uses to ignore these artificially created distractions can then be applied to the voices and used to deliberately tune them out.

8 *Dismissing the Voices*

Ordering the voices to go away or telling them to keep quiet sometimes helps people get free of their disturbing influence. A dismissal procedure which may be specifically effective for stopping critical or hostile voices involves the following simple steps:[448]

- In a loud and clear voice the hearer says: 'Go away and leave me alone!'
- The hearer adds strong emphasis to this command (e.g. by stamping their foot or pounding their fist on a tabletop as they command the voices to go away).
- If necessary the procedure can be repeated several times.

In order to be most effective this dismissal procedure should be done in a loud and clear voice with emphasis added. Some people may find that using somewhat stronger language is more effective (e.g. telling the voices to 'piss off!') When done as described it can help to enhance a person's sense of control. It also requires the hearer to utilise their vocal chords which in itself may help to stop the voices (see 'Vocal Activity' above). In order to avoid embarrassment or misunderstanding this method should generally only be used in private.

9 *Thought Stopping*

The technique of 'Thought Stopping' is often taught in stress management programmes as a tool to help people eliminate stress-producing thoughts (e.g. negative 'self-talk'). A method based on this technique might be useful to people who are troubled by persistent voices. A possible procedure is as follows:

• As soon as the voices begin the hearer says to them out loud: 'Stop!'
• The hearer immediately thinks of something pleasant, pays attention to the environment, and begins doing something to occupy their mind.
• If the voices persist the hearer should again say out loud, 'Stop!' and then try to create an image of something pleasant in their mind.

This procedure should be used as soon as the voices begin. In order to ensure its effectiveness the person using it must immediately turn their mind to something pleasant once they have ordered the voices to stop. After a while the 'Stop!' command can be whispered quietly rather than said out loud. Eventually, simply *thinking* 'Stop!' may be sufficient to eliminate the voices. As with the 'Dismissal' procedure described above some people may find that using somewhat stronger language will work better for them. The effectiveness of the 'Thought Stopping' technique may also be enhanced if a person snaps a rubber band against their wrist each time they order the voices to 'Stop!' (see 'Aversion Therapy' below).

10 *Aversion Therapy*

The rationale behind aversion therapy is that if an unwanted thought or experience is *immediately* followed by a painful or unpleasant consequence that thought or experience will eventually begin to occur less often. Researchers have used aversion therapy in an attempt to eliminate voices, e.g. by administering a painful stimulus such as a mild electric shock to a person whenever they begin to hear them.[449] A safe aversion therapy technique which can easily be self-administered involves a person wearing a thin rubber or elastic band around their wrist which they snap sharply against their skin the moment the voices begin. The pain this causes is quite harmless and it may eventually help to reduce the frequency of voices.[450] A variation on this technique involves the hearer merely *imagining* that some extremely unpleasant experience (e.g. severe pain, nausea, vomiting) will occur whenever they begin to hear voices. A significant reduction in voice frequency has been reported by some persons who have used these methods.

11 Self-Monitoring

This technique involves a person keeping a detailed on-going record of the occurrence, duration and content of their voice experiences. In order to do this they should carry a notebook and a pen at all times and every time the voices begin they should write down:

• When the voices started (the exact time of day – e.g. 11.44 p.m.)
• Where they were when the voices started (specific location – e.g. waiting at bus stop)
• What the voices said (the exact words used – e.g. 'Let's get him')
• How long the voices lasted (e.g. 9 minutes)

For this method to be most effective recordings must be made each and every time voices are heard and *as soon as possible* after they begin. A significant reduction in the frequency of voices has been reported by some people who have used this method.[451] (Note: As well as reducing voice frequency this technique provides information that may be very useful in helping a person to identify any specific situations that tend to 'trigger' the onset of their voices – e.g. certain times of day, particular locations, etc.)

12 Reasoning with the Voices

Voices are sometimes amenable to reason or can be bargained with. In such cases the hearer may be able to set certain limits on them. Sandra, for example, was able to free herself from the male voice she heard by coming to an agreement with him:

> I feel like there's a person inside of me, a male, and we talk to each other. Sometimes it goes on all day, we just talk as if he was walking beside me. But I've got a plan. I said to him, 'I'll see you after I die, and we'll meet at such-and-such a place.' I said, 'Now, we won't talk any more.

You don't talk to me, and I won't talk to you, and we won't annoy each other.' And he agrees to it.[452]

In some instances it may even be possible to 'timetable' the voices. For example, a person might try telling the voices that they will only listen to them at certain pre-determined times and will ignore them outside of these allotted periods. Voices sometimes accept this and agree to leave the person alone outside of the specified times. One woman gave the following description of how she managed to timetable her voices:

> I made a deal with the voices. After eight o'clock it is their time. I don't answer telephone calls and I don't meet other people from eight o'clock onwards. During the day they hardly bother me now and I am able to function much better in daily life.[453]

13 *Challenging the Voices*

To a large extent the power of the voices is determined by the identity given to them by the hearer. For example, if a person believes that a particular voice belongs to God, or to a spirit or some other kind of supernatural agency, they may feel quite powerless to oppose its demands or wishes. On the other hand, if a person believes that their voices actually originate from within (see 'First Person Singular' below), they are more likely to feel able to oppose them if that is what they choose to do. Research has shown that therapists are sometimes able to significantly undermine the apparent power and authority of voices by using an approach which involves systematically challenging the hearer's core beliefs about them.[454] Challenging the claims and identity of voices can be done in many different ways. Some of the following questions may help in challenging the voice's claims and identity:

- How are voices which claim to be supernatural agencies or entities (such as spirits) actually heard? Do they speak with *human* voices? If so, does this suggest anything about their true identity?
- If the voices make predictions, do the predictions always come true? If not, what does this say about their supposed power to accurately predict the future?

- If the voices claim to have special powers and abilities, what proof is there that they actually do? For example, one man heard voices which claimed to be able to read people's minds. He demanded that they prove that they were actually able to do this, and when it became clear that they could not, they left him alone.
- If the voices seem to be able to predict the future, is it possible that they are only echoing what the hearer might have known by other means? For example, a voice may predict that there will shortly be a knock on the door, but the hearer may have subconsciously heard someone walking up the driveway and therefore actually have been expecting to hear a knock at any moment.
- Are the voice's statements or commands consistent with their supposed identity? For example, does a voice which claims to be God or an angel encourage constructive and loving behaviour or does it have a negative and destructive influence?
- If the voices threaten dire consequences for disobeying them are the threats actually carried out? Many people who hear commanding voices are able to simply ignore their commands with no obvious adverse consequences.
- Despite their initial passivity many people discover that they actually have some ability to turn their voices on and off. For instance, some people learn that they can make the voices start by placing themselves in a situation which acts as a specific 'trigger' (e.g. a high stress situation), and they can use various coping strategies to make them stop (e.g. listening to music on stereo headphones). What does this ability to control the presence of voices say about their true nature and identity?

Just as they might rehearse what they plan to say at a meeting or interview well before it actually takes place, a person may find it helpful to decide what they want to say to the voices and practise saying it when the voices are silent. Then, if they begin the hearer will feel more confident standing up to them. Anyone who decides to challenge the voices should begin with their weakest beliefs about them first. For example, a person may be absolutely convinced that a particular voice is a spirit but have some doubts about its claims to be able to read minds. In this case they should first challenge the voice to prove its mind-reading ability. If the voice fails at this they might then go on to challenge the idea that the voice is actually a spirit. Challenging the voices can have the effect of diminishing their power and control and in some cases it may even make them disappear. (Note: Some people may find that their voices initially become *worse* when they are challenged. They may even threaten terrible retribution for daring to oppose them. Persistence in these efforts usually pays off eventually, however, and many people will find that in time their problems with voices begin to diminish.)

14 *First Person Singular Therapy*

This technique is based on the assumption that voices often originate in the hearer's own thoughts. According to this view, people who hear voices are actually talking to themselves without knowing it. By adopting the first person singular and consistently referring to their voices as 'me talking to myself' some people have been able to eliminate them. For example, a man who experienced high levels of stress whenever he had to make a difficult decision was helped in this situation by voices which told him what to do. This relieved his anxiety but also removed any sense of responsibility from him. He was encouraged not to refer to these experiences as 'my voices' but to call them 'my thoughts' instead. When he did this consistently for a short while the voices disappeared. Another example involved a woman who, during periods of painful loneliness, heard voices telling her how bad and unlovable she was. She was eventually able to realise that what she heard the voices saying to her was actually what she thought of herself. From then on, each time she heard the voices she said, 'I am telling myself I am bad and unlovable'. This resulted in the complete disappearance of the voices within a short time.[455]

15 *Selective Listening*

Many people who are troubled by critical or otherwise negative voices also hear others which they experience as being positive, helpful and good. For example, it is not uncommon for people living with schizophrenia to hear a mixture of benevolent 'higher order' and malevolent 'lower order' voices (these were discussed in detail in Chapter Seven). People who hear both positive ('good') and negative ('bad') voices may sometimes be able to deliberately ignore the negative ones and selectively focus their attention only on those which are positive. The positive influence that some voices can have was illustrated by the experiences of a woman who had tried ignoring all her voices at first, until she realised that some of them were actually helpful to her. Following this she listened and talked only to the positive voices, tried to understand the meaning of what they had to say, and cautiously accepted their guidance:

> In this period of ignoring the voices, to my surprise there were two voices that wanted to help me. My first reaction was to send them away, because this whole story was getting on my nerves, but they insisted that I needed them and to be honest, I realised this was true. The voices taught me how to watch, hear, and feel. For example, they asked me: 'How do you hear us and in what way do we talk to you?' And I, very smart, answered: 'Well, I just hear you with my ears, and you talk with your mouth.' 'Oh, really,' was the answer, 'then where is our larynx and in the same time we would like you to notice how you answer us.' I was very much amused by this last remark. At first I took everything literally which didn't improve the already strained relation with the voices. We then agreed to say everything twice, at least the important things: once as we always did, and the second time in symbols in an expressive way. The receiver would repeat the essence of what was expressed. At first we jerked along. I wasn't used to thinking in symbols at all, but I could immediately apply what they taught me and as a result I began to feel better.[456]

Though there is a generally prevailing view that *all* voices are indicative of 'mental illness' and therefore undesirable, some therapists believe that 'good' or 'helpful' voices can sometimes play an important role in assisting and supporting the hearer's psychological growth and emotional healing. (This notion is discussed more fully in the next chapter.)

16 *Cultivating Self-Esteem*

Disturbing voices sometimes begin to disappear spontaneously as a person's self-esteem improves. This is especially likely with respect to critical voices which often seem to reflect how a person is feeling about him or herself (see 'First Person Singular' above). Learning effective techniques to stop or control voices, such as the ones described in this chapter, may in itself contribute to improving a person's self-confidence and self-esteem as well as helping to reduce feelings of powerlessness. In addition, there are a number of quite simple methods that can be used to boost self-esteem. For example, repeating affirmations and consciously practising positive self-talk can be very effective. Marcia Lovejoy used affirmations to help herself get free of critical voices: 'I learned to write and then repeat to myself positive statements, which helped to dissolve the depreciating and frightening voices.'[457] Maryanne Handel also found that practising positive self-talk helped:

> I had to keep telling myself that I was a good person. I didn't think this out intellectually, but I kept saying to myself, 'I am a good person. There are lots of people who like me and lots of people who love me'. When I'd say these things the voices would just retreat and they'd fade away, as if I'd passed a test.[458]

Some people might find it helpful to write down a number of affirmations or make a list of their positive qualities and achievements which they then read to themselves several times a day as a form of self-therapy. In order for this to be really effective it is essential that the person reads the affirmations and positive self-statements with full attention to their meaning while trying to really feel their truthfulness. As a variation of this method a person could make a tape recording in which they say positive things about themselves (they could ask trusted friends or helpers to contribute some comments to the tape). If critical voices begin creating a disturbance reading the list of positive statements or listening to the tape recording can be very comforting and reassuring.

Long-standing problems with feelings such as anger, guilt, unworthiness, and inadequacy often play a significant part in the development of voices, especially those which are hostile and critical. Bottled-up fear or guilt can sometimes develop to the point where it may seem impossible to deal with; these feelings can then create the emotional turmoil which mental symptoms begin to feed off. In such cases counselling or other forms of therapy can be very beneficial. Although it may be difficult initially, the support of a trusted helper makes it easier to begin the process of getting feelings out into the open where they can be looked at and dealt with. Assertiveness training can also contribute to reducing problems with voices by helping a person develop confidence in their ability to express their true feelings and wishes.

17 *Maintaining Positive Attitudes and Expectations*

A person's expectation that they will hear voices sometimes seems to increase the likelihood that they actually will (the importance of the so-called 'listening attitude' was discussed earlier). On the other hand, people who believe that they can do something to actively prevent or control the voices sometimes find that this belief in itself seems to reduce their frequency. This fact was borne out by research designed to test the effectiveness of aversion therapy on voices.[459] In this experiment people with a diagnosis of schizophrenia were asked to use a portable electrical device to give themselves a mild electric shock each time they heard a voice. A third of the volunteers had a real 'shock machine' but another third had been given a *dummy* machine which they thought was giving them a mild shock but which actually did nothing. The remaining third of the volunteers (the controls) received no treatment for their voices during the experimental period. Members of *all three* groups reported having experienced a significant decrease in their voices during the two week trial! The fact that there were no major differences between the three groups led the researchers to conclude that the main factor that caused the reduction in voices was the so-called 'placebo' effect. In other words, people's *expectation* that participating in the experiment would help them with their disturbing voices actually caused this to happen.

Some people who have been troubled by voices gain significant relief by accepting their experiences and learning to think about them in a new and more positive way. As an example, a 30-year old woman living with schizophrenia heard voices giving her orders and forbidding her from doing things. Her life had become increasingly isolated and restricted by them and, though prescribed medication did not help, she was reassured to discover a new way of thinking about her voices. Her treating psychiatrist described how this came about:

> Last year she started to talk increasingly about suicide. I
> felt she was taking a road with no turning point. The only

positive topic in our communication then was the theory she developed about the phenomenon of the voices. The theory was based on a book written by the American psychologist Julian Jaynes, *The Origin of Consciousness in the Breakdown of the Bicameral Mind.* It was reassuring to her that the author described hearing voices as having been a normal way of making decisions until about 1300 BC. According to Jaynes, hearing voices has disappeared and been replaced by what we now call 'consciousness'. I began to wonder if she could communicate especially effectively with others who also heard voices, and whether her theory would be accepted by other people who had these experiences . . . She and I began to plan together how she might share some of her experiences and views.[460]

People who hear voices are often considerably relieved to discover just how common this type of experience is and how many well-known and highly influential people have had it in one form or another. In time many people who continue to hear voices are able to develop explanations for them which they are comfortable with and which enhance their ability to cope in a creative way. The development of a positive, accepting attitude can be helped enormously if a person is able to find a social or religious group in which their voice experiences are accepted and valued. Interestingly, a hopeful and positive attitude may do more than simply enhance a person's ability to cope with voices. Some research has shown that when people living with schizophrenia become more hopeful about themselves and their future prospects their distressing voices sometimes begin to be less dominating and may even fade considerably.[461]

18 *Restricting or Avoiding Non-Prescription Drugs*

The fact that voice experiences can sometimes be 'triggered' by illicit drugs (and possibly even by excessive consumption of social drugs) was discussed earlier. Since the possible effects of both these groups of substances is highly individual each person must discover for themself whether or not certain chemicals may bring on or worsen their voices. This requires a process of trial-and-error and careful self-observation. As an example of how this could be done, a person might try limiting their intake of caffeine, or even stopping it completely for a few days, in order to see if doing so makes any difference to their voices. A similar experiment could also be tried with alcohol and nicotine. It is worth keeping in mind that some common over-the-counter medications (e.g. some cold and flu remedies) may contain antihistamines or other drugs which might trigger voices in susceptible individuals. (See Chapter Three for further information about drugs and voices.)

People who have long-term problems with voices sometimes 'self-medicate' with various non-prescription drugs in order to reduce their anxiety and tension or to escape temporarily from their distress. Some people find that alcohol helps to relieve their disturbing voices and, even if drinking does not make the voices stop completely, it can sometimes cause them to change (e.g. the voices may become less attacking and more kind). Moderate alcohol consumption (i.e. up to two cans of beer, two small glasses of wine, or one ounce of spirits in any 24-hour period) is probably safe.[462] Caution must always be exercised, however, especially as the effects of alcohol can be exaggerated when consumed by someone who also takes prescribed psychotropic medication. This combination could cause drowsiness or impairment of coordination which may make it risky to drive a motor vehicle or operate machinery. Some people react adversely to even quite small amounts of alcohol and should probably abstain from drinking altogether.

In general, 'street drugs' such as marijuana ('pot', 'dope'), amphetamines ('speed'), and hallucinogens (LSD, 'magic mushrooms') are likely to lead to an increase in the occurrence and severity of disturbing voices. While some people claim to experience a degree of relief from voices when they use these drugs their effects can be extremely unpredictable. In some instances they may actually contribute to *worsening* a person's mental condition without them recognising that this is happening. A growing number of people who have been diagnosed as having a psychiatric disorder subsequently develop alcohol or drug abuse problems (a so-called 'dual diagnosis') as a result of attempts at self-medication which have gotten out of control.

19 *Psychotropic Medications*

Some people who hear voices have a psychiatric diagnosis. In such cases the voices are likely to be viewed as psychotic symptoms (i.e.

'verbal auditory hallucinations') which will either disappear or at least be brought under control as the diagnosed person receives effective treatment for their disorder. Neuroleptic medications are often prescribed to help control the symptoms of psychotic disorders such as schizophrenia, schizoaffective disorder, and bipolar disorder and are therefore classified as 'anti-psychotic' drugs. They may help to reduce or eliminate voices, although it can take several weeks before they reach their optimal effectiveness. Furthermore, since response to psychotropic drugs is known to be highly individual, it is sometimes necessary for a person to have a trial period on a number of different neuroleptic drugs or to experiment with different dosages of a single drug before the most effective regime is eventually found.

There continues to be considerable controversy regarding precisely how neuroleptic drugs work. There is little doubt that at least some of their therapeutic efficacy can be attributed to the placebo effect. Furthermore, although they are often referred to as 'anti-psychotic', in actual fact they probably do not have a specific effect on psychotic symptoms as such. This view is supported by the finding that a considerable proportion of people living with schizophrenia continue to hear voices (or experience other psychotic symptoms) despite the fact that they are taking neuroleptic medications as prescribed.[463] Rather than being specifically anti-psychotic the primary effect of these drugs may be to induce a feeling of 'not getting worked up' or a 'who cares' feeling. In other words, they have a rather non-specific calming effect.[464] Since voices are often 'triggered' by excessive stress and emotional over-stimulation such a generalised calming effect can be helpful in preventing them or at least diminishing their intensity. The calming effect of neuroleptic drugs can be especially valuable during an acute psychotic episode or if a person is feeling overwhelmed by threatening or attacking voices. Even if the drugs do not completely eradicate voices they often help to considerably reduce the hearer's anxiety about them. Thus, even though people on such medication may continue to hear voices, they often feel less troubled by them (e.g. 'The voices are still there but now I am able to just ignore them').

There are a number of important points that should be borne in mind regarding the use of neuroleptic drugs. Firstly, because it is still common for voices to be seen as a key symptom of schizophrenia, people who hear them are sometimes *inappropriately* diagnosed and treated for this disorder. This misunderstanding still occurs despite the fact that many people who hear voices do not have schizophrenia or any other kind of psychiatric disorder. Furthermore, some people who hear voices may have a disorder for which drug treatment is not appropriate. For example, people with multiple personality disorder (MPD) may be incorrectly diagnosed and inappropriately treated for years before the true nature of their problems is established. A second important consideration is the fact that, although they are generally given for their 'anti-psychotic' effects, neuroleptic drugs can sometimes *cause* voices or make them become worse.[465] Some people who take these drugs also experience considerable frustration at the fact that they are so non-specific in their effect that any 'good' voices they hear are just as likely to be eradicated as are 'bad' (disturbing) ones. This concern may lead some people to refuse these drugs.

Unfortunately, neuroleptic drugs have many potentially debilitating side-effects which can include depression, loss of motivation, numbing of emotions and dampening of creativity.[466] While the non-specific calming effect of these drugs can be extremely beneficial at times, a state of mental and emotional numbness ('psychic indifference') can result if this calming effect is induced to an excessive degree.[467] The use of practical coping strategies such as those outlined in this chapter may significantly reduce or even eliminate some people's need for neuroleptic drugs and thus minimise any problematic side-effects. In addition, it has recently been established that drugs belonging to the benzodiazepine group (i.e. so-called 'minor tranquillisers' such as diazepam) may sometimes be effective in helping to control voices.[468] Some people who have not responded well to neuroleptic drugs are reported to have benefited from treatment with these drugs. *It should be noted that drugs of the benzodiazepine group are potentially addictive and may therefore not be suitable for long-term use.*

20 *Miscellaneous Strategies*

With time and a little experimentation some people may eventually discover effective ways to stop or control their disturbing voices in addition to the ones listed above. People often develop highly individualised strategies for dealing with their voices. For example, one man discovered that he heard voices if he lay with his neck at a specific angle but when he shifted to a different position the voices stopped.[469] Some people find that devising personally meaningful rituals helps them to cope. Included among the very wide range of things that people have reported as having helped them with voices are: sleeping, eating ('comfort foods'), reading, dancing to lively music, playing with pets, prayer, reading the Bible, meditation, playing a musical instrument, sex/masturbation, psychic self-protection ('creating a circle of white light around myself'), adopting a more healthy lifestyle, and natural therapies (e.g. special diets, yoga, massage, herbal medicine, Reiki).

The Importance of Practice

Learning to cope with voices is a process that takes time. While the techniques described above can be learned quite easily by most people, as with any other kind of skill some practice is necessary. The following general suggestions may help to further enhance the effectiveness of voice-control strategies:

Modify the techniques

The coping strategies and techniques have all been described in very general terms so that they are easy for anyone to understand. However, their effectiveness may sometimes be increased if they are modified or adapted to suit an individual's specific needs and circumstances. For example, one person who used the 'Thought Stopping' technique found that saying 'Stop!' did not have the desired effect, but when he told the voices to 'Go to hell!' they left him alone. There is plenty of room for creativity, experimentation and ingenuity.

Use a combination of different techniques

Rather than using one single technique it is possible that a combination of two or more of them will often work best. As an example, a person could experiment with decreasing their intake of stimulant drugs (such as caffeine) *and* learning to use relaxation techniques *and* using affirmations to build up their self-esteem.

Use coping techniques that have already worked

Many people who have heard voices for some time may have already discovered through their own experience certain things that help. As long as these aren't harmful to anyone they should still be used. In some cases it may be possible to build upon or modify proven strategies using some of the practical suggestions outlined in this chapter.

Practise the techniques when not hearing voices

Most people will find it easiest to learn voice-control techniques when they are feeling good and are not being troubled by any voices. Then, if voices do occur again later on, they will begin their coping response with a greater sense of confidence in their ability to handle them.

Confront known 'trigger' situations

When a person has developed confidence in their ability to cope with disturbing voices they may feel ready to *deliberately* put themselves into situations which they know from past experience have tended to 'trigger' their voices (e.g. stressful situations). Doing this creates an opportunity to practise new skills in a situation which in the past may have seemed too difficult to handle. As an example, a man had avoided travelling on trains because doing so caused his stress levels to become too high and made his voices begin. He learnt an effective relaxation technique and found that, if he began using it as soon as he boarded a train, he could travel without being troubled by any voices.

Deliberately induce voices

Some people may be able to deliberately make their voices begin (e.g by placing themself in a 'trigger' situation). A person who is able to do this could use it to create a convenient opportunity in which to learn and practise coping strategies and techniques. In addition, if a person discovers that they have an ability to make their voices start and stop they will inevitably begin to see that they

actually have much more control over them than they may have
previously realised.

Life After Voices

Whether they are pleasant or unpleasant, voices often come to play
an important part in a person's life. Those which have been around
for a long time may have become such familiar 'companions' that
it can be hard to imagine not having them around any more. In fact,
it is not at all unusual for people to experience a sense of loss or
emptiness in their life if their voices do eventually disappear – even
if they have been predominantly negative! As strange as it may
seem, having problems can become a habit and some people
unconsciously create new problems to replace old ones that are no
longer there. Some people who have experienced disturbing voices
may sooner or later have to face the challenge of creating something
other than a new problem in their life when the old one has gone.
It is good to remember that choice is always possible: instead of
finding or creating new problems people can choose to devote their
energy to creating a better and more fulfilling life for themselves
and others.

Chapter Nine

LIVING WITH VOICES

Every complex, every psychic figure in your dreams knows
more about itself and what it's doing and what it's there for
than you do. So you may as well respect it.

— James Hillman[470]

The lives of many people throughout the world have been influenced in a positive and beneficial way because of the experience of hearing voices. In some cases this has occurred as a direct result of the inspiration, guidance, comfort and companionship which individuals have received from voices they themselves have heard; in others, though the beneficial effects may have come about in a more indirect way, they can nevertheless be traced back to an original voice experience. As an example, the lives of countless individuals have been spiritually enriched by the inspired teachings of saints and other religious figures subject to locutions. For millennia voice experiences of one kind or another have played a vital role in the daily lives of vast numbers of people in non-Western cultures (through such widespread practices as shamanism, for example). In the modern West a growing number of well-educated 'normal' people believe that it is possible to receive guidance, instruction or healing from various non-physical sources, some of which may communicate by means of inner voices (popular examples include channelling, spiritualism, and the near-death experience). Although scientifically acceptable proof is presently lacking, there is an impressive and rapidly expanding body of anecdotal evidence which suggests that, as long as appropriate guidance is followed and careful discernment exercised, such communications may indeed bring significant benefits to many people.

Given the fact that there is still often considerable fear and distress associated with voice hearing experiences many people may assume that, at the very most, the statements above could only apply to voices which have distinctly positive and helpful qualities, such as those which occur in a legitimate spiritual context, for example. This may not necessarily be the case, however. This chapter will consider the possibility that a wide range of voice experiences – including some which would ordinarily be classified as 'auditory hallucinations' and thus be made the focus of intensive efforts aimed at eliminating them – may have positive aspects and serve a range of useful purposes. Furthermore, it will be argued that some of these experiences undoubtedly have the potential to foster emotional healing and personal growth if they can be understood and worked with in a creative way. In light of such possibilities, rather than trying to get rid of voices, living creatively with them may be a feasible option for many people. In order to achieve this one of the most important prerequisites in many cases is a fundamental change of attitude.

Hallucinations or Voices? From Symptom to Experience

Some of the problems people have with voices (and with unshared sensory experiences generally) are exacerbated – if not caused – by the fact that they are feared. Indeed, it is no exaggeration to say that in some cases fear of the voices is itself the main problem! The persistent but *erroneous* belief that 'normal' people never have such experiences contributes significantly to this fear. People with a psychiatric diagnosis may be especially prone to developing negative feelings about voices since they are usually encouraged to think of them as psychotic 'symptoms', in which case hearing them may serve to constantly remind the person how 'sick' they are. In these circumstances it is hardly surprising that some people may eventually come to *hate* their voices. While this may be a very understandable reaction in some circumstances (such as when the voices are constantly hostile or critical) it sometimes occurs even though the voices themselves are not at all negative. As will be discussed later in this chapter, rather than being helpful such attitudes may actually contribute to making the hearer's problems significantly worse!

In order to explore the possibility of a more creative response it is first of all necessary to set aside all limiting and pejorative pathological terminology. Thus, rather than viewing voices as symptoms ('auditory hallucinations') and seeking ways to stop them, emphasis is placed on trying to understand them as a significant – if sometimes disturbing and disruptive – *inner experience*. It is worth remembering that until relatively recently people were never considered to be suffering from 'hallucinations'. Rather, they had *visions* (unshared visual experiences) and received *revelations* (unshared voice experiences). Whatever their ultimate 'cause' or combination of causes all voices – including those which occur in the context of psychiatric disorder – are an intimately personal experience whose roots are deeply embedded in the totality of the hearer's life and mind. This is true even if the voices have a substantial biological basis.[471] One eminent psychotherapist has explained why he adopts this kind of attitude toward his client's voice experiences:

> I accept my patient's experiences as simply human phenomena that are known to some extent by all of us, although their meanings may be obscure ... I avoid labelling my patient's experiences as exclusively patho-logic; rather, I am inclined to encourage him to accept them as a part of his life that should not be denied, even though it may be distressing and at times incomprehensible. All that exists outside our usual awareness is not to be avoided and feared as evil. We *are* our experience, and the dissociated (unfamiliar as it often seems to be) is a part of us and may be attended to with respect and profit; in it will be found wisdom as well as folly. In our waking imagery, in the dream, and in the hallucination exist elements of the accepting, unguarded spontaneity of the child and the creativity of the adult. Our therapy is directed at reducing the destructive consequences of anxiety. If our work goes well, the patient will have less to dissociate, and will come to be more at ease with imagination, the dream, and remem-brances of events now past and experienced in ways seemingly inconsistent with the adult's view of his culture.[472]

If an attitude of non-judgemental and tolerant acceptance is adopted by voice hearers and others – including any mental health professionals who may be involved – sometimes even quite frightening experiences may be remarkably transformed. In his book, *Awakenings*, the renowned neurologist Dr Oliver Sacks provides a graphic illustration of how this might come about. In the course of treating and caring for the last survivors of the great sleeping-sickness epidemic which swept the world in the 1920s, Sacks discovered that many of these long-institutionalised patients were 'chronic hallucinators'.* However, as a result of much time spent sensitively observing the specific effects the hallucinatory experiences had on the lives of these severely disabled people, Dr Sacks began to develop an accepting attitude towards many of them (an attitude that would have been very familiar to members of a shamanic culture!). He felt that the hallucinations of *some* patients undoubtedly served an important purpose and, as long as they remained under the person's control and were not being used to deny or escape reality, they represented a creative urge which ought to be accepted, perhaps even encouraged:

> I regard it as a sign of these patients' health, of their enduring wish to live, and live fully – if only in the realms of imagination and hallucination, which are the only realms where they still enjoy freedom – that they hallucinate all the richness and drama and fullness of life. They hallucinate to survive – as do subjects exposed to extreme sensory, motor, or social isolation; and for this reason, whenever I learn from such a patient that he constructs a rich hallucinatory 'life', I encourage him to the full, as I encourage all creative endeavours which reach out to life.[473]

The effects of Dr Sacks' accepting attitude were especially noticeable in the life of one particular person, Mrs Gertie C. Following treatment with the anti-parkinsonian drug L-dopa, this woman had started having 'visions' of a masked man outside the window of her hospital room (as described in Chapter One, an hallucinatory syndrome is a common accompaniment of long-term treatment of Parkinson's

---

* Sacks has emphasised that it took *many years* for these patients to trust him sufficiently to reveal their most intimate experiences and feelings to him. Only after they had known each other for almost a decade was he in a position to make the observation that at least a third, and possibly a majority, of the most deeply disabled and longest-institutionalised patients were, indeed, 'chronic hallucinators'.

disease with L-dopa). The presence of this man filled her with terror at first, but when he gave her a devilish grin her fear began to give way to unmistakable relish. When he appeared again, this time coming closer to her and flourishing his stick in a brazenly suggestive manner, she found herself developing warm feelings towards him and decided it was time to challenge Dr Sacks about it. His benevolent response helped to bring about a transformation in the quality of her mysterious 'hallucinatory visitor':

> On the third day Mrs C. decided to 'have it out' with me: 'You can't blame me', she said. 'I haven't had anything for the last twenty years, and I'm not about to get anything *now*, you know ... You surely wouldn't forbid a friendly hallucination to a frustrated old lady like me!' I replied that if her hallucinations had a pleasant and controllable character, they seemed rather a good idea under the circumstances. *After this, the paranoid quality entirely dropped away, and her hallucinatory encounters became purely amicable and amorous.* She developed a humour and tact and control – never allowing herself a hallucination before eight in the evening and keeping its duration to thirty or forty minutes at most. If her relatives stayed too late, she would explain firmly but pleasantly that she was expecting 'a gentleman visitor from out of town' in a few minutes time and she felt he might take it amiss if he was kept waiting outside.[474]

While on one level this woman's nocturnal experiences might appropriately be described as medication-induced 'hallucinations' they were nevertheless also an *experience* with substantial psychological and social dimensions. It was clear to Dr Sacks that in this particular case they had a positive and beneficial effect on the woman's mental state and contributed significantly to her state of emotional well-being:

> Mrs C. is alive and as well as she can be considering the severity of her illness. The deep peaceful look has returned to her eyes, and she seems to have regained her power for timeless contemplation of childhood scenes and moments. The only change in her from pre-dopa days is that she now receives love, attention, and invisible presents from a hallucinatory gentleman who faithfully visits each evening.[475]

Leonard L., another of Dr Sacks' patients who practised 'controlled hallucinosis', was able to confine his imagery to the blank screen of a television set or a picture which hung on the wall opposite his bed. For many years it had been his custom to 'animate' this particular painting for an 'hallucinatory matinee' every day after lunch.

Accepting and Listening to the Voices

The very idea of encouraging people to actively accept and listen to their voices – possibly even to speak with them – is likely to be greeted with considerable scepticism by many people, especially if the voice-hearers concerned have been diagnosed with a psychotic disorder such as schizophrenia. One very understandable concern is that this approach may seem to be encouraging a preoccupation with unreality and could therefore be seen as reinforcing maladaptive behaviour and dysfunction. Although certain risks may sometimes be involved – and for this reason a number of important precautions and safeguards should always be taken, as described below – it is nevertheless a fact that many people who hear voices feel they benefit in some way as a result of their contact with these invisible presences.

This is obviously true in regard to many 'normal' people who have had such experiences, as previous chapters have shown. Even among those who have a psychiatric diagnosis it may be true more frequently than is usually realised. As evidence of this a recent study revealed that among a group of psychiatric patients who had had various kinds of hallucinations including voices, *many* (52%) felt that these experiences had a number of positive effects including making them feel loved and providing them with companionship.[476] Indeed, many people said they would like to continue having these experiences if only they could learn to control them.* Sara Maitland's own voice

---

* The fact that some people choose *not* to use coping strategies which have proven to be effective suggests that they may be reluctant to lose their voices entirely. A high proportion of the participants in one study, for example, did not continue using practical coping strategies despite acknowledging them to be highly effective in making their voices stop (see Nelson et al., 1991). It may be that some people unconsciously resist losing voices which have developed from 'split off' and projected feelings and wishes (see Chapter Six) since these voices actually contain a 'lost' part of the hearer's own being.

experiences led her to develop a quite similar attitude:

> Clearly many people do find voice hearing very
> disturbing – but do all voice hearers want all their voices
> silenced at all times? Occasionally I would like mine
> silenced because they are frightening or just inconvenient,
> but equally they can be exciting, companionable,
> expressive, glorious ... I am not at all sure that I want
> them silenced – *especially* if they are an integral and
> internal part of an owned self, because silencing them
> would only be a further repression ... The voices would
> be even more useful if I could decode them better. What I
> want, far more than I want them silenced, is some skills in
> managing them. My voices seem to me to be very like
> having highly active and intelligent toddlers in the house:
> the exhaustion they cause does not mean you want them
> dead – it means you want them to behave better.[477]

Such attitudes are apparently not unusual. For example, when a
group of people living with schizophrenia were intensively
interviewed (each for a total of 30 to 40 hours) about voices which
had initially seemed to be mainly critical and hostile it was
discovered that the persecutory aspects represented only a *part* of
their actual experiences with the voices. Although persecution often
did occur the interviewees emphasised that the voices were mainly
helpful, beneficial and protective and that they frequently offered
advice, instruction and guidance. The researcher concluded that
many people probably withhold considerably the full extent of their
voice experiences, possibly because they often involve such private
and intimate feelings and relationships:

> For example, a patient to be described, at first, as was
> typical of most others, emphasised the persecutory aspects
> of her voices. However, later when her confidence had been
> gained, she described that her relationship with the voices
> was principally beneficial. For example, she believed their
> efforts were therapeutic ... They gave her direct advice
> such as not to tell others especially psychiatrists, that she
> heard voices ... There was, in addition, a complicated
> sexual relationship with her voices that was gratifying [and
> which] led to direct sexual discharge, a discharge that the

patient called an 'orgasm'. She explained that she was permitted to partake in the intercourse of male and female voices who were married and experienced their sensations as a 'third party'.[478]

It is easy to underestimate the richness and complexity of the relationships that many people develop with their voices. One clinical psychologist who researched this much-neglected area found that psychiatric patients had little difficulty using a standard questionnaire to rate their voices as if they were other *people*.[479] She discovered that those who had been hearing voices for some time often develop interpersonal relationships with them which involve many of the qualities of ordinary person-to-person relationships and that these relationships are often an important source of comfort and support. For example, one man with a diagnosis of paranoid schizophrenia said that his voice always lovingly looked after him, protected and backed him up, figured out and explained things to him, and taught him to understand and do things. It always paid close attention to him so that it could figure out all his needs and take care of them. This researcher commented that, while it may be a surprise to some to learn that a voice could be experienced as so loving and nurturing, this finding was not at all unusual. Even some of those who heard mainly hostile voices felt that the voices nonetheless liked them.

Voices which are hostile and antagonistic during the acute phase of a psychotic episode sometimes seem to spontaneously change and become more helpful and friendly as things begin to settle down again (i.e. as the person enters 'remission'). If this type of change does occur some therapists believe that it makes good sense to support the activities of such voices since they may actually be helping the diagnosed person to cope and adapt.[480] Although this suggestion is at odds with the usual approach which considers *all* voices, whether or not they are friendly, to be undesirable 'psychotic symptoms', a number of well-respected psychiatric authorities have argued in favour of it.[481]

After undertaking a comprehensive examination of a wide range of strategies for coping with disturbing voices two highly regarded clinical psychologists concluded that one of the most useful strategies of all involves deliberately focusing attention on the voices.[482] They surmised, furthermore, that the effectiveness of coping strategies such as self-monitoring, aversion therapy and first person singular therapy (described in Chapter Eight) may be largely due to the fact that they all require the hearer to focus on the voices.

Because deliberately focusing attention on hostile or critical voices is likely to be anxiety-provoking some therapists recommend that a graduated approach should be used.[483] For example, anyone who hears persistent disturbing voices could approach the task of focusing attention on them in a series of steps, beginning with attending to the voices' physical characteristics and gradually working up to a close examination of key beliefs about their identity and purpose. The person doing the exercise should go at their own pace and use their personal comfort level as a guide when working through these four successive steps:

(1) *Physical characteristics of the voices*

The hearer focuses attention on specific characteristics of the voices such as: the number of voices; their location; their gender (male, female, neuter); their ages; their vocal qualities (e.g. loudness, tone, accent). If there is more than one voice each should be focused on in turn (i.e. one voice at a time) until all voices have been accounted for.

(2) *Content of the voices*

Once the hearer is able to comfortably focus on the physical characteristics of the voices they should begin focusing on the content of what the voices say. Specific themes should be noted (e.g. threats, criticism, mockery) as well as the particular words, phrases and expressions they tend to use.

(3) *Related thoughts and feelings*

This involves the hearer paying close attention to any thoughts and feelings they have which are directly related to voices. Some of these thoughts and feelings may occur *after* hearing a voice (e.g. anger, fear, depression, negative self-talk) while others may occur immediately *before* the voices are heard (e.g. loneliness, self-criticism).

(4) *The meaning of the voices*

The hearer should attempt to identify the various beliefs they have about the voices (e.g. who or what the voices are, what their purpose is, what they want, why they are speaking at this time, and so on).

A person doing this focusing exercise should keep a detailed written record of their observations. Particular attention should be paid to any changes which occur in the frequency or quality of the voices while doing the exercise. As with some of the coping strategies described in Chapter Eight, this technique may work most effectively for some people if they do it with the support of a trusted and experienced therapist or counsellor. Although focusing attention on disturbing voices may lead to an increase in the hearer's anxiety in the short term, significant benefits may result over time. For example, it may become clear that some beliefs about the voices lack any real supporting evidence and need to be modified (e.g. the voices do not really have the powers they claim to have).

Some people who use the focusing technique may discover that voices which originally seemed to be coming from outside actually originate within them. Furthermore, while techniques which aim to suppress or distract attention away from disturbing voices pay no attention to their specific content, focusing can help the hearer gain new insights into how what the voices say relates to their frame of mind, self-esteem or current social situation, aspects of which are often reflected by the voice content (e.g. after an argument with her husband a woman heard the voices saying things about him which she was unable to bring herself to say). Some people who use focusing may become aware that the voices themselves are not particularly disturbing and that it is actually the feelings and thoughts they have about them which cause most of their distress. This is a potentially invaluable discovery because even if people are unable to stop the voices themselves they may nevertheless be able to modify the distressing thoughts and feelings they have about them (which in itself may lead to subsequent changes in the voices).

Deliberately focusing attention on disturbing voices may sometimes result in a significant change in their quality. For example, voices which were once hostile and threatening may start to become less aggressive and some may even disappear altogether. An illustration of this process can be found in the experiences of a man in his early sixties whose voices started when he was in his late teens and continued unabated for the next forty years despite the fact that he received a wide variety of psychiatric treatments. He heard three or four different voices but the most persistently troublesome was one he identified as that of the choirmaster of a church choir he had sung with when young. He remembered this man as having always picked on him for not singing the right notes. Over the many years he heard voices he had never been encouraged to talk about them let alone *to* them, but one day he decided to do just this:

> [On] this particular day he decided that he was going to talk to the choirmaster. He addressed the man saying that he had always enjoyed singing as a youngster, and he often wished to join a choir again. That could be arranged, replied the choirmaster, and the next day he started to hear a choir singing his favourite hymns and chorales, so he joined in. After a couple of days' membership of this hallucinatory choir, he suddenly decided to stop singing, and he angrily told the choir to go away. The following day the choirmaster returned, demanding to know why he hadn't been turning up to rehearsals. The gentleman replied that he had decided to leave the choir because he was fed up with the other members who were singing out of tune. He added that as far as he was concerned he was fed up with the choirmaster's criticism over the years, and he too could get lost. He never heard the voice again.[484]

If focusing on voices leads to them becoming less troublesome a state of harmonious coexistence with them may become a real possibility for the first time. As an illustration of this, Professor John Strauss has described how the voice experiences of a young man with a diagnosis of schizophrenia changed over time as a result of his cultivating a more tolerant and accepting attitude towards them:

> At first he felt the voices were entirely hostile since they threatened and made fun of his efforts to get ahead in life and to reach his goals of success. Increasingly, however, he found that it was not possible merely to ignore or argue down these voices, or even to capitulate to them. Rather,

he attempted increasingly to negotiate with them, to take them seriously, and to come to some kind of 'modus vivendi' with them. This young man ... already finds this negotiation seems to allow him to progress further with his ambitions than had been possible previously. He is hopeful ... that this approach may help him to succeed where before he had met only with increased intensity of his voices and with failure, frustration, and relapse.[485]

Focusing attention on voices and listening carefully to what they say is an *experiment*. As such it should be done in a spirit of curiosity and with an open-minded attitude. As with any experiment it is not possible to predict in advance exactly what might happen. Consequently, some common-sense guidelines should always be followed:

- Focusing may not be suitable for all people who hear voices. It is specifically *not* recommended for people with a psychiatric disorder who are still acutely disturbed. Such people may find some of the coping strategies described in Chapter Eight more useful until they have regained their emotional and psychological stability and become more 'grounded'.
- Ideally this type of experiment should be conducted with the support and guidance of trusted, sensitive and experienced helpers.
- Listening to voices does *not* necessarily imply believing everything they say or doing whatever they command!
- It is very important for a person to always keep their feet firmly planted on the ground. Keeping up with ordinary activities and responsibilities in the everyday world and seeking feedback from others will help to minimise any risk of becoming 'lost' in the world of the voices.
- Relationships with inner voices may exist alongside those that are maintained with ordinary people in the everyday world: they should never become a substitute or replacement for relationships with ordinary people.

A Meaningful Disturbance: Learning From the Voices

From what has been said so far it is clear that rather than continuing to struggle desperately *against* the voices that disturb them some people living with schizophrenia may be able to find ways of understanding and working creatively *with* them. Maryanne Handel's experiences provide a graphic illustration of this possibility. In the course of a painful struggle to be rid of the hostile male voice which had tormented her for over two years this young woman made a number of discoveries which eventually led to a remarkable transformation, not only in the voice itself, but in her life as a whole. Looking back, she made the following summary observation regarding her struggle:

> I think the worst thing is to be afraid of it. One shouldn't resist it or try to squash it or be afraid of it because it's not going to work. It will never go away if you do that. I used to ask this voice to go away but it would never go away when I wanted it to. It doesn't work like that. It only started to go away and eventually went away when I had changed, and when I felt better about myself and who I was and when I felt better about this voice and that it wasn't trying to hurt me.[486]

It is possible to glean many valuable lessons from the complex transformation process Maryanne Handel underwent. Her experiences suggest that the process of learning from disturbing voices involves at least four interrelated aspects which can be divided as follows:

(a) Facing the Fear of the Voices
(b) Accepting the Voices as an Inner Experience
(c) Attributing a Meaning and Purpose to the Voices
(d) Relating to the Voices in a Different Way

(a) Facing the Fear of the Voices

If a person hears voices which seem to be totally negative and destructive all they may want to do is get rid of them or get away from them. Although this is a very understandable reaction anyone who wishes to explore the possibility of gaining something of value from their voice experiences must try to control their fear and overcome their desire to escape. A person undoubtedly needs a great deal of courage to begin facing voices that have become like 'scary monsters' which constantly threaten and attack. Facing such voices often requires a person to confront personal issues which are threatening and anxiety-provoking. For example, Maryanne Handel discovered that the critical male voice she heard had its origin in her own deeply ingrained feelings of self-disgust and self-hatred and that she needed to deal with these feelings before she could regain her peace of mind and begin moving forward in her life.

While people frightened by hostile or critical voices may be very reluctant to deliberately focus attention on them, as was explained in the previous section it is sometimes very helpful to do precisely this. In some cases focusing attention on the voices may even make them stop.* On the other hand, constantly trying to *avoid* the voices may sometimes have the effect of maintaining them.[487] It not clear why this should be so, although many people have probably had experiences (not necessarily related to hearing voices) in which the very act of running away from some feared person or situation sometimes seems to actually create the 'monster' from which they are trying so desperately to escape! In such cases the 'monster' may continue to be frightening until the fleeing person finds the courage to stop running away and begins dealing with the situation that originally caused their fear.

In Chapter Eight a number of general suggestions were made which may be of use to anyone struggling with their fear of voices. There are no easy answers or 'quick fixes', however, and in the end each person must find their own way of dealing with fear. Maryanne Handel found that it helped to keep telling herself that all the strange things she was experiencing were part of a test she was required to undergo:

> I knew that fear would be my worst enemy and I had to
> not be afraid of anything I heard or felt. I wasn't brought
> up to believe anything in particular but I'd read bits and
> pieces from the Bible and things came back to me, phrases
> like 'perfect love casts out fear'. And I kept saying these

---

* This possibility was noted by Eugen Bleuler, the Swiss psychiatrist who coined the term schizophrenia. Professor Bleuler stated: 'It can happen that taking notice will obliterate the hallucination.' (Bleuler, 1950, p.108). The eminent psychopathologist Karl Jaspers also noted that sense-deceptions will sometimes disappear 'if full attention is directed upon them' (Jaspers, 1963, p.141).

things to myself because I had to ward off fear. One night when I had all these visions and hallucinations come up to me I remembered once hearing some sort of legend, a story about a man who had to go and spend a night in a ruined temple. He was told that there would be all sorts of demons and phantoms, evil things that would come and visit him in the night, and that what he had to do was not be afraid of anything he saw. This was his sort of test. And I thought, well, what I am going through is sort of like that. I have to not be afraid of anything I see, no matter what it looks like. And so I didn't. No matter what it looked like or said, I made myself not be afraid.[488]

People who can contain their fear and resist the urge to flee may sometimes discover that hidden among the 'bad' voices there may also be some 'good' and potentially helpful ones. Closer scrutiny may even reveal that there is another 'side' to voices which had previously seemed totally negative and destructive (as discussed below, even apparently 'demonic' voices sometimes seem to have benevolent qualities). In this regard voices sometimes seem to be rather like certain people who, while they may be quite nasty at times, nevertheless often have a softer and more 'human' side – although it may be kept very well hidden!

(b) Accepting the Voices as an Inner Experience

Many people who hear voices recognise from the very start that they are not hearing the voices of other people and that this experience takes place only on an inner level. Such voices are 'heard in the mind' and have been variously referred to as 'loud thoughts', 'thoughts becoming audible' and so on. On the other hand, many people are quite convinced, at least initially, that the voices *do* originate in some location outside of themselves (e.g. from other people, hidden loudspeakers, the spirit world). A significant step towards developing a more creative approach involves the hearer coming to understand that, no matter where the voices *seem* to be coming from, they are actually an *inner* experience. In other words, hearing voices is a private perceptual experience which is not shared by others. In this regard it could be compared to dreaming since dreams, too, are a totally private, inner experience even though they often involve hearing sounds (auditory perceptions) which seem to be coming from somewhere outside of the dreamer.

The inner nature of voice experiences may be very difficult for some people to accept at first – especially if the voices seem to be speaking loudly enough for other people nearby to also be able to hear them! Anyone who thinks that their voices do actually emanate from an outside source might like to consider the following ideas. Firstly, just because the voices *seem* to be coming from outside does not mean that they actually are (remember what happens in dreams). Secondly, if the voices were coming from an outside source other people in the vicinity ought to be able to hear them too. Given this, anyone who hears voices could consider asking other people nearby if they can also hear them. If these people say they cannot, then one of the following three explanations is possible: (a) These people are lying; (b) The voices are being directed specifically at the hearer in such a way that other people cannot hear them; (c) The voices are an inner experience. Weighing up the pros and cons of each of these possibilities may help some people become clearer about the inner nature of their voice experiences.[489]

Once they are able to accept that their voices are a private perceptual experience a person might begin considering the possibility that they actually originate from within their own mind (in 'self talk', for example). In considering this idea it is important for the hearer to remain open to the possibility that the voices may come from some part of themselves they are (currently) unaware of. For example, Maryanne Handel has described how for a long time she had been totally convinced that the voice which tormented her was that of a man she had once worked with, but she eventually came to realise that 'he' actually represented a part of herself (her conscience):

> One day I decided to call it my conscience and so I'd say it was my conscience. Eventually I realised that it wasn't this other man's voice and I worked hard to understand that it never had been. Eventually I could see that it never had been him although it always looked like him in my mind and it always sounded like his voice. It still went on but I could see that it was sort of an impersonal voice and not his voice. It always felt like it was not me, like it was

something or somebody else, it felt foreign, not me. But eventually I came to see that it was from within me. It still felt sort of foreign, but I could feel that it was not from outside anyway. I knew that and so I eventually gave it that name.[490]

The process of learning to accept voices as an inner experience is sometimes very difficult, especially with regard to voices which originate in disowned and projected memories, 'split off' feelings, and unaccepted aspects of the hearer's self-image (see Chapter Six). In such cases the task of learning to see the voices as part of oneself often requires the hearer to acknowledge and come to terms with his or her *personal* 'demons' and 'angels', as Rachel Corday has explained:

It is not as though we have been invaded by beings outside ourselves, from other realms or planets, angels trying to help us or demons trying to destroy us. We have our demons and angels within our own consciousness.[491]

(c) Attributing a Meaning and Purpose to the Voices

The meaning and personal significance of an experience is not simply given but is *attributed* to it by the experiencer. In other words, it is what a person makes of an experience that will determine its real meaning for him or her. For this reason the beliefs that a person holds about the voices they hear play a very important role in determining how they will respond to them. For example, if the hearer is convinced that the voices are a punishment or a malicious attack by powerful unseen external enemies they may feel vulnerable and powerless to do anything other than attempt to escape. If the voices are taken to be an unequivocal symptom of 'insanity' their presence may be very frightening and demoralising, both to the hearer and to others. Similarly, anyone who believes they are besieged (or even possessed) by 'evil spirits' may feel overwhelmed by hopelessness and despair. On the other hand, attributing a constructive meaning and purpose to the voices can help to open up the possibility of a range of creative and even growth-promoting responses to them.

Those inclined to think of voices only as psychotic 'symptoms' may have considerable difficulty accepting that they could ever serve any constructive purpose. It is interesting to note, therefore, that Professor Eugen Bleuler was of the opinion that the voices heard by people living with schizophrenia sometimes represent 'well-founded criticism of their delusional thoughts and pathological drives.'[492] He also noted that 'sensory deceptions may represent ... that part of the personality which has remained normal with regard to its critical faculties and possibly its partial insight'.[493] On the basis of his own clinical observations Carl Jung also formed the impression that the voices of even the most severely disturbed individuals may sometimes have a constructive purpose. For example, he believed that despite the severity of their condition such persons often retain a 'normal' personality which 'stands looking on in the background' and which may, by means of 'correcting voices', sometimes make entirely sensible remarks and objections:

> It is remarkable that not a few patients who delight in neologisms and bizarre delusional ideas ... are often corrected by their voices. One of my patients, for example, was twitted by the voices about her delusions of grandeur, or the voices commanded her to tell the doctor who was examining her delusions 'not to bother himself with these things'. Another patient, who has been in the clinic for a number of years and always spoke in a disdainful way about his family, was told by the voices that he was 'homesick'. From these and numerous other examples I have gained the impression that the correcting voices may perhaps be irruptions of the repressed normal remnant of the ego-complex.[494]

Further insight into these possibilities can be gained by examining the specific content of voice experiences. Although in most clinical settings little attention tends to be paid to what the voices actually say, the particular things a person hears may sometimes reveal a great deal about their social and emotional state. It is not unusual for voices to express hopes or longings that, for one reason or another, the hearer feels unable to express more directly: 'Wounded wishes find a home in hallucinations.'[495] At the beginning of the century Professor Bleuler noted that the voices heard by persons diagnosed with schizophrenia 'embody all their strivings' and 'express ever the same wishes, hopes and fears'.[496] Following his own in-depth study of psychotic and religious experiences the founder of pastoral psychology, Anton Boisen, reached the conclusion that it is very important to pay attention to the specific content of voice experiences:

> Voices and other hallucinations indicate a stirring of the deeper levels of the mental life, something which in itself may be helpful as well as destructive. Their chief significance lies in what they may reveal as to the inner trends and attitudes. What the voices say is always the important question, not the mere fact of hearing voices.[497]

The content of the voices' utterances often tend to focus around a few specific themes. It is very common, for example, for voices to make references to the hearer's sexuality, relationships, and self-image. In such instances the voices may actually be serving the purpose of reflecting some aspect of the hearer's current social or emotional state which could potentially provide them (and others) with valuable insights into some of the specific issues or conflicts they need to deal with. For example, people who are berated by voices which accuse them of being a totally inadequate failure are very likely to have significant problems with self-esteem which they need to address. (In Chapter Seven the view was put that the purpose of so-called 'lower order' voices was to illustrate and make conscious the hearer's weaknesses and faults, while voices of the 'higher order' possibly reflected their unrealised potentials.) Though it may be distressing to hear, what the voices say may sometimes be at least partially true. For example, one woman was troubled by a voice which kept saying things like, 'You don't care for anybody else', 'You just care for yourself', 'You don't love anybody, you just pretend to love'.[498]

The focusing exercise described earlier can help a person gain insight into the meaning and significance of what the voices say. As a result of her own prolonged struggle Maryanne Handel gradually developed a new understanding of the purpose of the voices which attacked her. After finally accepting that they actually came from within her she began to think of them as having been sent to teach her something. She used this explanation to reassure herself whenever she felt under attack:

> I'd start to instinctively feel afraid, and then I'd start to

think, 'What are they doing to me?', and then I'd think to
myself, 'No, no', and I'd make myself calm down and I'd
say, 'No, nobody's trying to hurt me, it's allright, nobody
even wants to hurt me, they're just trying to show me
something. It's like a test'. And if I calm down I can control
it, then if I survive the test I feel stronger. They are just
trying to make me feel stronger.[499]

Eventually she concluded that the frightening, attacking voices were
actually a reflection of her own inner emotional state:

These very threatening, ugly, unpleasant hallucinations and
voices and instructions (I was told to kill myself) made me
feel that I deserved to die, I had to die. But I still believed
that they were trying to teach me something and so it began
to mean something to me. All these images suggested to
me something about me, about my state, about what I
thought of myself. It was like they were saying to me,
'Look, this is what you really think of yourself!' If you
have all these horrifying, negative things coming at you
like I did, well it seems to me that if it comes from within
you, from your own subconscious, it must mean something
about what's within you. All the voice's anger and
contempt and hatred seemed to correspond to feelings and
thoughts I had about myself. So I think that is what has to
be changed. That is what is within you and it will only
change and go away when *you* change.[500]

Voices sometimes seem to serve a fairly obvious purpose. For
example, they may provide welcome and valued companionship to
someone who is lonely and isolated. (Even critical voices may
sometimes serve this purpose. As Oscar Wilde once noted, the only
thing worse than being talked about is *not* being talked about!) Their
possible meaning and purpose often tends to be rather obscure,
however. One of the main factors that contributes to this is the
tendency of voices to use highly symbolic forms of communication.
For instance, voices might speak about 'light' and 'dark' in
reference to love and hatred, or they may say that something is
'poison', meaning that it is bad for the hearer not that it is actually
physically poisonous. (It is not clear why voices communicate in
this particular way any more than it is known why dreams are so

symbolic.) In many cases the specific meaning of the voices' utterances may remain totally incomprehensible until the hearer stops taking them literally and begins to understand them metaphorically, just as they might do when trying to decipher the meaning of dream symbols or the lines of an obscure poem. The first major breakthrough in John Perceval's struggle with voices came with the dawning of this realisation: 'I suspect that many of the delusions which I laboured under, and which other insane persons labour under, consist in mistaking a figurative or poetic form of speech for a literal one ... '[501] Since it is ultimately the hearer who attributes a specific meaning to the words spoken by voices their meaning is often highly idiosyncratic. Sometimes a short phrase or even a single word will communicate something of great personal significance to the hearer.[502] One of Maryanne Handel's experiences provides a good illustration of this:

> After the voice had become less aggressive it started to say things to me, it would confirm or deny thoughts I'd had, and I began to see there was a kind of pattern to it. For example, if I had a certain kind of thought or made a certain kind of statement it would say 'exactly so'. I couldn't understand this at first and it went through different phases, but at a certain stage whenever I'd have some terribly negative, horrible thought about myself or other people or about life, the voice would say to me 'exactly so'. At first I thought it was telling me that what I had been thinking was true, but after a while I began to see that every time I had a really destructive thought and the voice would say 'exactly so' it was confirming, not that it was true, but that I'd had a really bad thought. Sometimes on other occasions when I'd had some thought that was more constructive and true, the voice would say 'just so', very quietly. I began to see a pattern because every time it said 'just so', that's when I'd thought something good and positive, but when it said 'exactly so', that's when I'd thought something rotten. I could see that it was sort of like a guidance, that it was telling me what kind of thoughts I was having, so I began to change those and to consciously make myself have more positive thoughts.[503]

The task of developing a set of beliefs about voice experiences which will help to reduce the hearer's anxiety at the same time as attributing some constructive meaning and purpose to them may be helped by the following:

• Considering a range of different theories regarding the nature and origin of voices. (A number of these were described in Chapter Six.)
• Discussing voice experiences with sensitive and empathic helpers who are open to some of the possibilities discussed in this chapter.
• Meeting with and talking to other people who have heard voices.
• Reading about the many different ways voice experiences have been interpreted. (A list of Recommended Reading can be found at the end of this book.)

(d) Relating to the Voices in a Different Way

It is understandable that people who feel attacked, ridiculed, criticised or controlled by voices often feel very angry toward their invisible tormentors. 'Why are they doing this to me?' and 'Why don't they just go away and leave me alone?' are questions such persons frequently ask. While they may eventually learn to tolerate persistent critical voices many people nevertheless harbour feelings of resentment toward them, and some even indulge in secret wishes for revenge. Although such feelings may seem perfectly justified to the victim of unprovoked attacks, they may actually make matters worse since hostility and anger directed at critical voices can have the effect of 'adding fuel to the fire'. One woman gave an example of how this can occur: 'I argued with the voices. So we scolded each other; there was a lot of negative communication. This only made the voices stronger and more aggressive.'⁵⁰⁴ Dr Edward Podvoll, a psychiatrist who has made an intensive study of Eastern approaches to psychosis, has suggested an alternative which he believes is more likely to result in an enhancement of the hearer's peace of mind. Thus, instead of trying to retaliate against hostile other-worldly voices, Dr Podvoll believes that it is far better to cultivate a compassionate attitude toward them:

> Aggression toward the other world is basically aggression toward one's own mind; it cannot help but have negative effects. If there is to be a genuine turning away from the

other world it can only be done with an attitude of light-handedness and gentleness. The Tibetan medical tradition takes this notion much further: when someone feels he is suffering under the influence of 'beings' in the other world he is advised to be compassionate toward them because they only attack him out of their own misery.[505]

Many religious and spiritual traditions advocate a similar attitude. In the New Testament, for instance, the advice is given: 'Love your enemies, do good to those who hate you, bless those who curse you, pray for those who abuse you.' (Luke, 6:27–28) Some people have found that it helps to apply this advice to 'unseen enemies' which come in the shape of attacking or critical voices. Maryanne Handel has described how developing a loving attitude toward the voices which tormented her eventually brought about a total transformation in her situation:

> If you think that somebody is trying to hurt you or hates you, what you should do is put out loving thoughts to this person in your head. You don't even have to say it outwardly in words, but in your mind what you have to do is put out kind, generous, loving thoughts. You say in your mind nice things about this person. I did this whenever I saw these images or heard this voice: I would be nice to it, kind to it, and I would think good thoughts about these people and who they were and it really helped. It made me feel better, and then all these hallucinations and voices would just begin to retreat and get softer and fade.[506]

Some people who feel tormented or intruded upon by voices may feel that they could never forgive them, let alone 'love' them. It is worth remembering in such cases that it takes at least two parties to create and maintain a state of conflict. Some people may find that if they can simply 'drop' any anger and resentment they feel toward the voices the vicious circle of escalating hostility and antagonism will be broken. Following this new discoveries may sometimes be made about the voices' purpose and nature. For example, when a hostile voice is finally given an opportunity to be listened to the hearer may discover that it has previously unrecognised qualities and needs. In some cases the voices may even complain about the fact that the hearer never listens to them or takes them seriously.[507] In this regard the behaviour of voices sometimes seems to resemble that of the hostile persecutor 'alter' personalities which trouble people with multiple personality disorder (MPD). One authority on MPD has concluded that even though they act tough (some even identify themselves as demons or other powerful supernatural beings), hostile alters really just want to be loved. Often, he believes, their hostility is a way of concealing their pain and sadness: 'They are often adolescent but may claim to be demons, dead relatives, or other figures. They often present as tough, uncaring, and scornful, but this is usually just a front for an unhappy, lonely, rejected self-identity.'[508]

As with hostile 'alter' personalities it may be that some attacking voices only *seem* to be evil and destructive because they are not understood and accepted. This is especially likely with respect to voices which have developed out of the hearer's rejected feelings, memories or wishes (see Chapter Six; for a discussion of the possible psychological origins of 'evil spirits' see Chapter Seven). In such cases, if the hearer can learn to accept them as being a necessary part of their whole self, an extraordinary metamorphosis may sometimes occur. The German poet Rainer Maria Rilke believed in the possibility of a transformation brought about through acceptance:

> How should we be able to forget those ancient myths that are the beginnings of all peoples, the myths about dragons that at the last moment turn into princesses; perhaps all the dragons of our lives are princesses who are only waiting to see us once beautiful and brave. Perhaps everything terrible is in its deepest being something helpless that wants help from us.[509]

In some cases, what was once experienced as an 'inner demon' may be transformed in a process that one Jungian therapist has likened to a kind of *psychological* exorcism:

> That is true exorcism: to accept everything in oneself that one is ashamed of before the eyes of the world. By doing this, one pins the demons down where they can do the least harm and where they are able to transform – and in this way casts them out.[510]

As described above, the male voice which had initially been

extremely hostile and critical toward Maryanne Handel gradually became softer and gentler as she sent it 'loving thoughts'. As she came to accept it and listened more closely to what it had to say a further transformation occurred which had a number of beneficial effects on her personality and general adjustment:

> The whole tone of the voice became softer and gentler, and after a while I could see that it sort of guided me. It reflected my relationships with other people in the real world and I began to change those consciously, making myself have more positive thoughts about other people, real people that I knew. I began to develop better relationships with people. It made me more aware of other people too, more understanding of their problems and less judgemental than I used to be, and less afraid of other people. It made me think a lot. It made me feel things and change things. It made me think also about other people and what they've been through. And it made me understand that really we have many problems in common.[511]

Many MPD therapists rely upon 'good' alter personalities in their work and some even try to recruit so-called 'internal self-helpers' as peers or even co-therapists.[512] In a somewhat similar fashion therapists sometimes find that they can help their clients most effectively if they endeavour to work *with* rather than against their voice experiences. As an example, Carl Jung has described how his therapeutic approach with an elderly woman who had lived with schizophrenia for many years was actually guided by one of her voices. This particular voice, he believed, represented the 'normal' aspect of her personality which continued to exist 'in the background' despite the severity of her psychiatric condition:

> She heard voices which were distributed throughout her entire body, and a voice in the middle of the thorax was 'God's voice'. 'We must rely on that voice', I said to her, and was astonished at my own courage. As a rule this voice made very sensible remarks, and with its aid I managed very well with the patient. Once the voice said, 'Let him test you on the Bible!' She brought along an old, tattered, much-read Bible, and at each visit I had to assign her a

chapter to read. The next time I had to test her on it. I did this for about seven years, once every two weeks. At first I felt very odd in this role, but after a while I realised what the lessons signified. In this way her attention was kept alert, so that she did not sink deeper into the disintegrating dream [of psychosis]. The result was that after some six years the voices which had formerly been everywhere had retired to the left half of her body, while the right half was completely free of them. Nor had the intensity of the phenomena been doubled on the left side; it was much the same as in the past. Hence it must be concluded that the patient was cured – at least half-way.[513]

The clinical psychologist Wilson Van Dusen (whose research was discussed in Chapter Seven) encouraged people with benevolent 'higher order' voices to accept and be guided by them. Although some of his patients were initially frightened by the apparent power and wisdom of these voices, some eventually benefited from accepting and integrating their spiritual qualities and values into themselves:

One patient described a higher order spirit who appeared all in white, radiant, very powerful in his presence and communicated directly with the spirit of the patient to guide him out of his hell ... Higher order hallucinations have [said] that they can control the lower order ones, but it is seldom to the degree the patient would desire. In some respects they overcome the evil in so far as the patient identifies with them. In one case I encouraged the patient to become acquainted with these helpful forces that tended to frighten him. When he did so their values merged into him and the evil plotters, who had been saying for months they would kill him, disappeared.[514]

Because there is always a possibility of deception great care should be exercised by anyone considering accepting the guidance of voices – even if they seem to be benevolent. *The guidelines for discernment outlined in Chapter Seven provide a simple and reliable safeguard which will help to minimise the likelihood of the hearer or others being led astray.*

Amplifying the Voices

As described above it is sometimes possible for a person to relate to or work with their voices in a way that enhances their peace of mind and which, in some instances, may even result in significant personal growth. This is especially likely if the voice experiences themselves are relatively simple and uncomplicated. However, because they often use highly symbolic forms of communication, the identity of the voices and the meaning of their utterances frequently remains obscure. In such cases there are a number of techniques which may help to clarify the situation so that a deeper understanding of their personal significance becomes possible. In some ways this approach could be compared to the various ways in which dreams can be worked with in order to unlock their richly symbolic creative potential.

The technique of *active imagination* developed by Carl Jung may sometimes be useful in working with voices to foster a rapprochement with them and clarify their personal meaning. In essence active imagination involves a person consciously entering into a dialogue with some aspect of themselves they wish to gain greater understanding of. The starting point could be a dream image, a feeling or mood, a physical symptom, a spontaneous fantasy, or an inner voice. The person doing active imagination simply focuses attention on the chosen image and then speaks with it and listens carefully to everything it says in response. This process is referred to as active imagination because it involves a person *actively* entering their inner psychological world in order to deliberately engage with the 'persons' (i.e. personified images) that are to be met there. When active imagination is used to work with voices it is as if a dialogue were taking place between two people, each of whom has a valid point of view. Such imaginative meetings might involve all of the familiar transactions that occur in everyday encounters between ordinary human beings: confronting and arguing, making friends, exchanging points of view, and learning from one another:

> In your imagination you begin to talk to your images and interact with them. They answer back. You are startled to find out that they express radically different viewpoints from those of your conscious mind. They tell you things you never consciously knew and express thoughts that you never consciously thought. Most people do a fair amount

of talking in their active imagination, exchanging points of view with the inner figures, trying to work out a middle ground between opposing views, even asking for advice from some very wise ones who live in the unconscious.[515]

It is very helpful for the person doing active imagination to write down everything they say and everything they hear in reply. This should be done even if what the voices say seems to be meaningless and nonsensical. The reason for writing everything down is that doing so helps to give a concrete reality to experiences that may otherwise easily become vague and confused. It also creates a permanent record which can be looked back on later when its meaning may be clearer. Some therapists encourage the use of painting, drawing, sculpting or clay modelling in conjunction with active imagination since these media allow aspects of inner experiences to be portrayed which may be difficult or even impossible to express in words.

Jung emphasised that at its most fundamental level active imagination represents an inner dialogue between the ego or conscious self of the participant and various personified aspects of the unconscious. Although at times these unconscious aspects may seem strange or frightening (just as the images appearing spontaneously in dreams sometimes do), they are nevertheless symbolically very meaningful. As such, even unwelcome images may have great personal significance:

> Through active imagination it becomes more and more clear that the images that appear in imagination are in fact *symbols*, representing deep interior parts of ourselves. Like dream images, they symbolise the contents of our unconscious. Because these interior beings have 'minds of their own', they say a do things that are new to us – startling, often enlightening, sometimes offensive to our egos.[516]

In the example that follows an approach based on active imagination was used to work therapeutically with a young man's disturbing voice experiences. In this particular instance the inner dialogue technique was augmented by the use of clay modelling. The person concerned was a nineteen year old man named Joe who was readmitted to hospital complaining of feeling controlled by Teresa, a young neighbour girl of fifteen whose voice he constantly heard. Joe had been given a diagnosis of schizophrenia and his treatment on previous occasions had involved individual therapy and medications to control his psychotic symptoms, although these had only been partially effective. The voice content was mostly sexual in nature and very distressing to Joe, who simply wanted Teresa to leave him alone:

> She talked to him in his ear, she breathed for him, she took blood from the sole of his foot and would not return it, she took his sperm, she shook his head, she made his hands do all sorts of crazy gesturing at inappropriate times, she made him see things that weren't there, she even masturbated him ... She incessantly wanted sex with him, was always filling his mind with sexual ideas and comments about himself and others and shouted obscenities in his ear. She would not leave him alone. He wanted to stop all this and complained of being weary of being her puppet. He wanted nothing to do with her, resented this constant sexual battering and wanted to be rid of her.[517]

Because the Jungian therapist who worked with Joe was only available for a limited time (they worked together for seven one-hour sessions over a three week period) he decided to focus each session primarily on the voices. From the very beginning of therapy Joe was asked to take note of everything Teresa said:

> I gave Joe a notebook in which to record dreams and everything the voices said between sessions. Occasionally, Teresa would say something during a session and Joe would tell me and these too were recorded. Every effort was made to get Joe to tell me and write down everything that was said by the voice. During the session, we would go over in great detail the things she had said, clarifying what was meant or referred to. My attitude was accepting, non-judgemental, and non-interpretive in relation to this material.[518]

In order to discover what Teresa might represent on an inner emotional level Joe's therapist felt that it was important to explore other aspects and dimensions of her identity. To begin this process he used one of the basic techniques of active imagination to help amplify her presence and make visible some of her other qualities. Since Joe's previous attempts to get rid of Teresa's voice only seemed to increase her power over him he was encouraged to try relating with her instead. The first step in this process involved getting him to approach her in fantasy. Interestingly, Teresa's controlling nature began to soften and transform as Joe moved away from being her passive victim:

> In our second session I asked Joe to close his eyes and visualise Teresa. He did this and quickly had an image of her. Only her head appeared at first followed later by the rest of her body. She was wearing a white dress and standing near a fence near her home. I asked Joe to approach her. He did so and said hello to her. In the fantasy she seemed quite shocked and was speechless for a long time. She finally said hello, smiled, got on a bicycle and rode off singing.[519]

A little later Joe was given some modelling clay and invited to make an image of Teresa. He did this and then proceeded to make a clay figure of himself. With the therapist's support and encouragement Joe used these clay figures to act out a fantasy in which he attempted to satisfy Teresa's sexual demands. Joe was very pleased with this work and it prompted a long and detailed discussion of his sexual concerns, ideas and memories. Following the therapy session in which Joe fantasised about sexually satisfying Teresa he was surprised when she unexpectedly revealed to him that she was a 'Mass' and could give 'Massing'. Joe told his therapist that she meant the Catholic Mass. This new image of Teresa as a 'priestess' stimulated a flood of memories relating to Joe's early experiences in the Catholic Church. One particularly powerful memory involved a time when Joe had gone to confess to the priest about masturbating but was unable to speak when he entered the confessional. It was the last time he ever went to confession.

Joe was quite perplexed at the emergence of a 'religious' side to Teresa, especially since her previous behaviour toward him had been blatantly sexual. However, his therapist recognised the significance of the fact that Teresa's religious side had only emerged *after* he had satisfied her sexual demands in fantasy using the clay figures. Although Joe was reluctant to hear what Teresa brought to him – sexuality and religion combined in one person –

his emotional healing seemed to require that he hear it. The revelation of her function as a priestess was a symbolic reflection of the bringing together of Joe's spiritual yearnings and his conflicted sexuality and lack of connection with his body. As such it heralded a decisive step forward in his psychological development:

> Teresa carries the secret of initiating the body into life, that is, into sexuality. For a young man particularly, sexuality forces him into life and therefore into separation from the mother ... The voices and visions of Teresa brought the reality of the body to Joe in a very forceful, unpleasant, and negative way. Rejecting her only brought more power to her. Teresa seemed to personify all that Joe wanted consciously to reject. Yet she now appears as a priestess able to give him the Mass, and thus becomes a mediator through which he could partake of a new spirit ... Taken in this way we are led to the hypothesis that some instinctual aspect of the feminine is the basis or origin of the voices and visions of Teresa. Moreover, it would be contact with the instinctive feminine – in this case Teresa – that could function to mediate and heal the splitting of Joe's personality. It was this contact with the image of Teresa in fantasy and in clay that characterised our work together.[520]

Joe was able to leave hospital shortly after the completion of these therapy sessions. Just before he left he told his therapist that he felt very pleased because Teresa was no longer bothering him so much. He went on to attend college where he majored in forestry.

In addition to its possible therapeutic use in amplifying disturbing voices so that the hearer may be able to learn something of value from them, the technique of active imagination can also be used to contact and dialogue with 'positive' inner voices. As a person cultivates a relationship with this aspect of themselves they may discover that such voices sometimes provide helpful insights and advice. At times they may even act as a source of inspirational guidance regarding important life decisions:

> Of course it can also be a positive voice we hear and with which we learn to talk. Just as there is a negative voice that seems to want us to fail in life, so there is a positive voice that gives us helpful insights and flashes of inspiration. We

can cultivate a relationship with this side of ourselves by learning to dialogue with it, and talk over with it our life situation. The ancients used to call such a figure a 'spiritus familiaris'. Socrates referred to it as his 'daimon', meaning not 'demon' in the negative sense of the word but his 'genius' or inspirational spirit. In Christian parlance it is a version of the guardian angel or a manifestation of the guidance of the Holy Spirit.[521]

In using active imagination to amplify and enter into dialogue with inner voices a number of precautions should always be observed. First and foremost, this kind of work should always be undertaken with great respect for the power of the unconscious. It is always advisable to have the on-going support and guidance of a trusted and experienced therapist or counsellor. This safeguard is especially important if previous experience has indicated that there is a possibility of a person becoming overwhelmed or even temporarily taken over by the voices. Anyone who does active imagination should immediately cease all such work and concentrate fully on getting themselves 'back down to earth' if they feel they are becoming overly anxious or being drawn excessively into their inner imaginal world. Jung himself emphasised how extremely important this is. In his autobiography he explained how his professional identity and responsibilities, family obligations, and other personal commitments in everyday reality helped him to remain 'grounded' during those times when he was engaged most intensively in exploring the mysterious world of his fantasies and inner voices:

It was essential for me to have a normal life in the real world as a counterpoise to that strange inner world. My family and my profession remained the base to which I could always return, assuring me that I was an actually existing, ordinary person. The unconscious contents could have driven me out of my wits. But my family [and the facts of my everyday existence] were actualities which made demands upon me and proved to me again and again that I really existed, that I was not a blank page whirling about in the winds of the spirit . . . I aimed, after all, at *this* world and *this* life. No matter how deeply absorbed or how blown about I was, I always knew that everything I was experiencing was ultimately directed at this real life of mine. I meant to meet its obligations and fulfil its meanings.[522]

Anyone who uses active imagination or some other technique to dialogue with inner voices should never lose sight of the deeper purpose of this challenging work. As Jung pointed out, establishing a relationship with voices is not done for its own sake. Rather, this undertaking should be seen as part of a much larger task in which a person strives to bring the many different parts of him/herself into closer and more harmonious relationship in order that they may progress toward discovering their true identity and rightful place and purpose in the world.

HEARING VOICES HAS OPENED MY EYES

The psyche is the greatest of all cosmic wonders and the sine qua non of the world as an object. It is in the highest degree odd that Western man, with but very few – and ever fewer – exceptions, apparently pays so little regard to this fact.

– Carl Jung[523]

I first started researching voices several years ago while writing a book I hoped would be a useful practical guide to understanding and coping for people living with schizophrenia. I had expected that it would take a few pages to describe the experience of 'auditory hallucinations' and outline some possible coping strategies. As I worked my way through the few books and articles I could find I very soon realised that they were not going to provide satisfactory answers to my many questions. Even more challenging was the fact that when I took the time to speak with people who actually heard voices they often described experiences which were very poorly accounted for in conventional textbooks – if they were mentioned at all! Increasingly I began to feel both frustrated and intrigued for I knew that I would never be satisfied until I had made a sincere attempt to develop an understanding that would do justice to the wide range of experiences that real people actually have with voices. As I continued my research I found myself being led off the familiar and well-worn path I'd trodden with countless others into what for me was new and totally unexplored territory. I gradually learnt to accept the strange mixture of fear and excitement that is familiar to anyone who approaches the limits of their understanding and contemplates what may lie beyond these comforting yet restricting boundaries.

The Clinician's Illusion

Like many others who work in the mental health field I had long believed that hearing voices must invariably be a frightening, disturbing and essentially negative experience. This is certainly what I had been taught. I also imagined that most people who hear voices would be desperate to get rid of them and that they would often be prepared to go to great lengths to do so. Furthermore, I thought that most people who hear voices 'suffer from schizophrenia' and – fortunately for them – that their voices could usually be controlled if not entirely eliminated by administering appropriate doses of neuroleptic medication. As I continued my research into the actual experience of hearing voices I started to realise for the first time how narrow and excessively negative my established views had been, although I had been completely unaware of the fact.

As my beliefs gradually changed I began to reflect on how I had formed such attitudes in the first place. Several influences soon became obvious. Firstly, it is a fact that people are most likely to report voice experiences to mental health professionals if they are troubled by them and want help. Consequently, professionals can easily form the impression that people who hear voices are *usually* troubled by them and want them to stop. It then becomes easy to overlook the fact that many people hear voices but don't complain about them simply because the voices themselves are not a problem. Among those who have been given a psychiatric diagnosis the existence of 'good' voices is also likely to be under-recognised because people generally only tell treating personnel about voices if they are disturbed by them. Because of this many mental health professionals are quite oblivious to the fact that human beings generally – including some who have a psychiatric disorder – are capable of having voice experiences which are positive and beneficial.

Another important influence that shapes attitudes toward voices is the fact that, although such experiences are actually quite common, fear and stigma cause many people to hide them from others. At the very least a person who admits to hearing voices runs the risk of being accused of 'hearing things' – if they are not considered to be 'mental'. Such fears have contributed to the fact that even now, at the beginning of the twenty-first century, we still have very little reliable information about the true prevalence of voice experiences in the human population. Even among those who *already* have a psychiatric diagnosis and who are acknowledged to hear voices a number of factors may conspire against open discussion of their experiences. For example, such people may deny the fact that they are still hearing voices because they wish to appear 'well'. Furthermore, psychiatric patients who hear friendly or helpful voices may choose to conceal their existence in order to avoid being given drugs which they fear will make them stop. In some cases there may even be subtle forms of 'punishment' meted out to patients who admit to hearing voices. Such punishment may come in the form of increases in medication, withholding of leave or discharge from hospital, or possibly even a less appealing diagnosis – schizophrenia is highly likely to be diagnosed if voices are prominent. Taken together these influences contribute to the impression that hearing voices is generally a disturbing experience and that it is relatively rare, except perhaps among persons with a diagnosis of schizophrenia (who are often thought of as the classic voice-hearers), especially those not taking neuroleptic drugs.

Listening to the Voices of Experience

The first of many challenges to my long-held beliefs came with the fortuitous discovery of a paper by Professor Marius Romme which described a congress organised for people who hear voices. In 1986 Professor Romme and one of his patients, a woman living with schizophrenia, discussed her voice experiences on a Dutch television talk show. Viewers who had also heard voices were invited to contact the station and 450 people did so and subsequently completed a questionnaire in which they described a very wide range of experiences with voices, some of which were positive while others were felt to be distressing or disabling in some way. A large proportion of the respondents claimed never to have sought or received any form of psychiatric treatment. From among those who had completed a questionnaire twenty people were selected and invited to be speakers at an inaugural 'Voice Hearers' Congress' held in October 1987 and attended by 300 people who heard voices. Reading an account of the Congress proceedings made me realise for the first time the extent to which my beliefs about voices had been almost exclusively founded upon a pathological perspective:

> The general atmosphere of the entire congress was of a meeting of a group of people with common interests and experiences. Although medical aspects of these experiences were discussed, there was no sense that this was a medical meeting or a meeting of medical patients. The participants freely shared their experiences, their many interpretations of these experiences including religious views or a range of other human reactions, and their approaches to coping. Some people were obviously troubled by their voices and saw them as part of a mental illness, but many had very different ways of understanding these experiences and appeared to be competent, not disabled, and depending on one's view of the nature of voices, not in any way 'ill'.[524]

Many of those attending the Congress interpreted their voices as guides, gods or spirits, people they knew, or as some kind of special gift. Some were troubled or disturbed by the voices and felt them to be a negative factor in their life. Professor Romme noted that 'hearing voices does not seem to be limited to psychiatric patients' and suggested, furthermore, that the wide range of experiences that people can have with voices calls for a much broader approach to them:

> One hypothesis that might be generated from this congress is that the reduction of 'hearing voices' to being viewed merely as a pathological phenomenon is not very fruitful in helping patients to deal with these experiences. It may also be inaccurate. Outside the world of psychiatry, many people hear voices and are quite able to handle them, even experiencing the voices as enriching their lives.[525]

As well as encouraging me to begin thinking in a far broader, less pathology-focused way reading about the 'Voice-Hearers' Congress' stimulated my curiosity to learn more about voice experiences. Thus began a personal and professional odyssey which has resulted in a deepening of my respect for the mysteries and complexities of the mind and a greater awareness of the profound importance of spirituality in human life.

Rethinking the Word 'Hallucination'

The experience of hearing voices is often classed as a type of auditory hallucination. According to one widely accepted definition an hallucination is 'A sensory perception that has the compelling sense of reality of a true perception but that occurs without external stimulation of the relevant sensory organ.'[526] As it is ordinarily used this term generally implies a pathological phenomenon – a sensory *deception*. As the disorders described earlier clearly show there are certain circumstances in which human beings *are* sometimes subject to various kinds of sensory deception. For example, a psychotic person may hear people talking about him or her when they are not in fact actually doing so. Nevertheless, the manner in which the word hallucinations has come to be understood and used has a number of unfortunate consequences. Most importantly, since it is based on a strictly materialistic view of the world it makes no allowance for the possibility that it might sometimes be quite normal for human beings to have vivid sensory experiences in the absence of an external physical stimulus. (Dreams are an obvious example of this.) If the conventionally accepted definition is applied St Teresa's locutions, the voices of childhood companions, bereavement experiences in which the deceased person is seen or heard, and many of the other kinds of experience described in this book would all be classified as auditory hallucinations. Once experiences are so labelled it becomes difficult to avoid the implication that the person having them is, by definition, deceived or mistaken (in keeping with the original meaning of the root word *alucinari*, 'to wander in mind'), and that their perceptions are inherently false or distorted.

The labelling of all unshared sensory experiences as hallucinations and the implication that it is *always* abnormal to see or hear things when nothing is physically present has many potentially untoward consequences. For example, the vivid sensory experiences which often occur as a helpful accompaniment of bereavement, or the voices which occasionally mediate spiritual revelation, may give rise to needless fear and anxiety in persons concerned about their sanity because they have been led to believe that such experiences cannot be 'normal'. It is also possible that the problems of people with a mental disorder such as schizophrenia may be exacerbated if it is not recognised that hallucinations may sometimes have positive effects (e.g. 'good' or 'higher order' voices). The existence of strongly negative attitudes about voices and other subjective sensory experiences may even have the effect of making them less likely to occur, which would be unfortunate in regard to experiences which may potentially be enjoyable or beneficial. At the beginning of the twentieth century Francis Galton's pioneering research (see Chapter One) led him to recognise that the tendency to experience voices and visions was not rare among human beings, but that it was often repressed in response to negatively judgemental social attitudes:

> The visionary tendency is much more common among sane people than is generally suspected. In early life, it seems to be a hard lesson to an imaginative child to distinguish between the real and visionary world. If the fantasies are habitually laughed at or otherwise discouraged, the child soon acquires the power to distinguish them; any incongruity or nonconformity is quickly noted, the visions are found out and discredited, and are no further attended to. In this way the natural tendency to see them is blunted by repression. Therefore, when popular opinion is of a matter-of-fact kind, the seers of visions keep quiet; they do not like to be thought fanciful or mad, and they hide their experiences, which only come to light through inquiries such as these that I have been making.[527]

It is quite clear that under certain circumstances human beings are capable of having vivid sensory experiences in the absence of a tangible external physical stimulus without any deception taking place. However, the English language presently lacks a word other than hallucination, with its accompanying implications of pathology and aberration, to refer to such experiences. A number of possible alternatives have been suggested. For example, the term 'benign hallucinations' has been proposed in the hope that the addition of the word 'benign' might signify that the experience is a fortunate or salutary one, or at least that it is not negative or malignant.[528] Another suggestion has been to confine the use of the word 'hallucination' to unshared sensory experiences which occur in the context of mental disorder and to use a new term (such as 'idiophany' – which literally means 'private appearing') to refer to all sensory experiences that arise in the absence of external, physical stimuli, including those which are not in any way pathological.[529]

These suggestions involve much more than merely playing with words. In fact, they call for a different way of looking at the world, one in which the value of a person's lived experience takes precedence over any attempt to judge, label and classify it. They also call for an openness to the existence of realms of experience beyond the physical. For these reasons they are likely to meet with considerable resistance. Nevertheless, until more appropriate terminology is devised it may be best to avoid pejorative terms such as 'auditory hallucinations' and to simply refer to the auditory verbal experiences which occur in the absence of tangible external stimuli as 'voices' or some such term, thereby avoiding any implication that they are necessarily pathological phenomena or symptomatic of a pathological state or condition.

Exploring the Realms of Non-Ordinary Perception

The understandable desire of people to conceal the fact that they have had experiences such as hearing voices contributes to the reinforcement of what is an already over-emphasised materialistic view of the world. It also makes it difficult to study such experiences in a rigorous and scientific manner. As a result, relatively little is known about them – except perhaps in circles which lie well outside the psychological and scientific mainstream. It is rather ironic that during the past century a great deal of the most important research into voice experiences has been conducted by those interested in parapsychology. Professor Sidgwick's innovative research on behalf of the Society for Psychical Research (described in Chapter One) is undoubtedly one of the important landmarks in the history of scientific attempts to investigate non-physical sensory phenomena.

Few people realise that among the pioneers of paranormal research, which began in earnest at the end of the nineteenth century, were some of the most eminent scientists, psychologists and philosophers of the day. Professor Sidgwick's interests were shared by sensitive thinkers of the calibre of William James (the 'father' of modern psychology), Carl Jung (founder of Analytical Psychology), Sigmund Freud (founder of Psychoanalysis, whose interest developed toward the end of his career), Sir Oliver Lodge and Sir William Crookes (scientists), and Arthur Conan Doyle (the writer who created Sherlock Holmes). In spite of their impeccable academic reputations and unquestionable sincerity, the authors of the seminal 'Census of Hallucinations' found very little support among their professional colleagues:

> At the Second International Congress of Experimental Psychology, held in London in 1892, Professor Henry Sidgwick read an abridgment of the Report, and in the discussion that followed, members of the Congress appeared to hold the view that anyone experiencing a hallucination of the human form must, *ipso facto*, be in a morbid state, although there is nothing in the Report to indicate this. There does not seem to have been any appreciation on the part of the psychologists present at the Congress of the theoretical importance of the work which the Census Committee had performed.[530]

In response to the materialistic bias that appears to have already been firmly entrenched in the minds of their fellow students of human behaviour the pioneer researchers eventually created a specialised field of study separate from conventional psychology – that of 'parapsychology'. The prefix 'para' alludes to the fact that the phenomena under investigation are *beside* or *beyond* those that constitute ordinary human experience (as well as being beyond the interests of conventional psychologists!) While parapsychological research has undoubtedly made many extremely valuable contributions to our understanding of the nature of non-physical perception it could be argued that the creation of a separate category for phenomena such as ESP, telepathy and clairvoyance has helped reinforce the view that they do not belong within the scope of *normal* human psychological functioning. It may be that this has inadvertently contributed to maintaining the cultural taboo which discourages open discussion of this realm of experience.

Within academic circles it takes considerable courage to declare an interest in 'psychic phenomena' (let alone to admit to believing in them!) This is a rather curious state of affairs since it is clear that one does not have to actually believe in the reality or existence of something in order for it to be a legitimate subject of study. After all, an atheist might find it extremely fascinating to study the psychology of religious belief systems in order to gain an understanding of how and why others hold the beliefs they do. Although it is probable that relatively few voice experiences involve genuine paranormal phenomena (see Chapter Six) a thorough study of this whole area is certainly intellectually and scientifically legitimate. One psychiatrist who holds this view has made the following observation and plea to his colleagues:

> The exclusion of extrasensory perception (ESP) from serious mainstream psychiatry is an artifact of our cultural history. There are only two possibilities concerning ESP experiences: Either they are real or they are illusory. If ESP is real, excluding it from psychiatry and mainstream science is prejudice masquerading as science. If ESP is not real, there is no more reason to exclude it from phenomenological study than any other set of delusions, including Schneiderian first-rank symptoms.[531]

It is heartening to note that there has been a resurgence of professional and lay interest in these matters over the past two decades. A particularly important development is the advent of Transpersonal Psychology, a broad field whose central concern is in understanding the nature and role in human life of experiences which transcend the boundaries of the ego and the limits of time and space. Having recognised the limitations inherent in conventional materialistic and egocentric approaches a growing number of psychologists, psychiatrists and other therapists have begun exploring the transpersonal perspective.[532] Carl Jung was one of the first psychologists to intuit the existence of a dimension of the human psyche that transcends the ego and many years of clinical observation and experience convinced him of its importance. Thus, after grappling with complex questions regarding the nature of 'spirits' and other occult phenomena, Jung finally concluded:

> After collecting psychological experiences from many people and many countries for fifty years ... I doubt whether an exclusively psychological approach can do justice to the phenomena in question. Not only the findings of parapsychology, but my own theoretical reflections ... have led me to certain postulates which touch on the realm of nuclear physics and the conception of the space-time continuum. This opens up the whole question of the transpsychic reality immediately underlying the psyche.[533]

On the basis of his extensive clinical experience and incisive scholarship the psychiatrist Stanislav Grof, one of the leading authorities in the burgeoning field of Transpersonal Psychology, has devised an 'extended cartography of the psyche' which recognises that normal human beings have a capacity for a much wider range of non-ordinary experiences (including voices and visions) than has previously been thought possible. Grof especially emphasises that the distinction between experiences which are potentially growth-promoting and those which are pathological lies more in the context in which they occur, the manner in which they are approached, and the ability to integrate them into everyday life, than in the intrinsic nature of the experiences themselves.[534]

Re-Visioning Psychiatry

Many people who hear voices are eventually given a psychiatric diagnosis and receive some form of medical treatment. Such interventions are obviously valuable if they help persons so diagnosed to feel more comfortable in themselves and foster their ability to function at an optimal level and move toward achieving their desired goals in life. While it is undoubtedly true that some people benefit considerably from conventional psychiatric treatment a number of trends have become increasingly influential in recent years which raise concerns about the quality and effectiveness of the help that people who hear voices are likely to receive from the mental health system.

Pre-eminent among the various influences that shape the views now held by large numbers of mental health professionals is the widespread ascendancy of biological psychiatry. In distinct contrast to trends evident in health care generally in which the importance of *holistic* approaches is increasingly emphasised, mainstream psychiatry has become almost exclusively focused on the search for the supposed biological causes of various mental disorders. Coupled with this there has developed a heavy reliance on physical methods of treatment, psychotropic drugs in particular. The views of biologically-oriented researchers are heavily promoted in both popular and academic publications despite the fact that critics of psychiatry's biological reductionism continue to point out the lack of a firm empirical basis for many of its claims.[535] Some professional journals have become so biased toward biomedical orthodoxy that those who do not subscribe to it may find it impossible to have their opinions and research findings published. It has also become increasingly difficult for researchers to secure adequate funding for work which does not emphasise biological considerations.

These trends have had a number of important ramifications for persons hearing voices who find themselves being treated within the orthodox mental health system. First and foremost, such persons are likely to be told that their voice experiences are symptoms of a mental illness which has a biological basis. Furthermore, they are likely to be prescribed 'anti-psychotic' (neuroleptic) drugs designed to control or eliminate the voices. In short, it is common for people to be told that a 'chemical imbalance' in their brain is responsible for causing psychotic symptoms such as auditory hallucinations (i.e. voices). These approaches may have a number of positive aspects. For one thing their extreme simplicity makes them easily under-standable by persons whose emotional distress may impair their ability to comprehend more complex information. Most importantly, the use of neuroleptic drugs often provides rapid and significant relief from the anxiety caused by disturbing voice experiences (as well as ameliorating other problems), thereby alleviating the distress of both the diagnosed person and others concerned, such as relatives and friends.

Despite these potential benefits it is increasingly apparent that the widespread acceptance and implementation of systems of mental health care based upon a simplistic biological model has significant disadvantages. For example, it is now commonplace in most psychiatric treatment settings for voices (and other experiences deemed to be psychotic) to be viewed as some kind of 'biologically driven craziness' which needs to be suppressed with medication. One unfortunate consequence of this approach is that people who hear voices are often given little opportunity to discuss their experiences in detail with the mental health professionals who are responsible for providing care and treatment.* (Economic constraints and other factors often further exacerbate the situation

---

* The recent advent of self-help groups (such as 'The Hearing Voices Network' – see Appendix) which aim to provide psychiatric service users with a safe, supportive environment in which they can share their voice experiences with others, can be seen as evidence of widespread disenchantment with the psychiatric status quo.

by pressuring staff to serve increasingly large numbers of clients with ever-diminishing resources.) The consequences can be dire. One group of people with first hand experience of this situation have described the frustrations it frequently gives rise to:

> Over the many years of our different connections with psychiatric services we have found little opportunity to speak openly of our day-to-day experiences of the voices and visions that have been so troublesome to us, or, for that matter, the voices and visions that have been helpful to our lives. We have been silenced time and again by many psychiatric professionals who have consistently refused to acknowledge our experiences of these voices and visions. At times we have been bewildered by this, at a loss to understand it. At times we have linked this silencing to the fear we see in the eyes of others ... At other times we understand that others believe that to make space for us to talk more openly of our experiences of troublesome voices and visions is counterproductive. We know that still others are caught up in weird theories about our experiences, and talk about our lives in ways that subtract from our sense of self-respect and make it impossible for them to hear what we have to say about our experiences of voices and visions.[536]

Mental health services which fail to create a climate in which people feel free to speak openly about their experiences may inadvertently contribute to exacerbating the emotional distress of clients and hamper their efforts to cope more effectively:

> Needless to say, this silencing has profoundly negative consequences to all of our lives. All of us have felt abandoned because of this. We have not felt joined with by others at those times in our lives when this was what we have longed for most. At times this very silencing has contributed to a sense that we might be going mad. And it has made it virtually impossible for us to change our relationship with the troublesome voices and visions that have been dominating our lives, and, as well, with the voices and visions that have been more supportive of us. We just cannot here emphasise strongly enough how

important it is to have the opportunity to speak of the troublesome voices and visions in a forum that contributes to a powerful exposé of their purposes and their operations ... This exposé disempowers them, and opens up possibilities for us to become much more aware of the knowledges and skills that we have that we can put to work to frustrate the attempts of the voices and visions to capture our lives.[537]

Since the effectiveness of drug treatment often tends to be measured primarily in terms of whether or not the voices (or other 'psychotic symptoms') are still present, biological psychiatry generally places little importance on their specific content (i.e. who the voices are and what they say). However, even if it were to be shown that some voices *do* have a substantial physical basis in the brain (as biological psychiatrists argue is the case with schizophrenia), voice content is nevertheless highly individualised and often reflects important personal concerns of the hearer, such as their conflicts regarding relationships, self-image, and sexuality (see Chapter Four). Ignoring voice content in treatment risks conveying a message to the hearer that his or her personal concerns are irrelevant or unimportant. Furthermore, failure to identify and deal with the client's significant personal issues increases the likelihood that treatment will be incomplete or possibly even ineffective. At the very least, avoidance of open discussion of voices (and other subjective phenomena) impairs the ability of helpers to empathise since to do so requires that they have a detailed and accurate knowledge of their clients' actual lived experience.

Excessive emphasis on biology may lead to a situation in which there is a real danger that the training of mental health professionals will no longer adequately equip them to respond in an effective way to the full range of their clients' psychological, social, emotional and spiritual needs. In this regard it is thought-provoking to reflect on the fact that the ancient Greek word 'psyche', from which modern terms such as 'psychology' and 'psychiatry' are derived, was originally understood to refer to the human soul or spirit. Although the term 'psychopathology' is often taken to be the study and classification of psychiatric symptoms (e.g. auditory hallucinations), its literal meaning is 'suffering of the soul'. The origin of this word reflects an appreciation of the fact that profound suffering can touch the core of our being. It also points toward the possibility that some symptoms may originate in the depths of the soul. Though it is seldom realised today, the word 'psychiatry' literally means 'the healing of the soul'.

Abandoning the Concept of Schizophrenia

It is instructive to compare contemporary biological orthodoxy with the views of the person who introduced the concept of schizophrenia to psychiatry. The Swiss psychiatrist Eugen Bleuler (1857–1939), whose stature within the field of psychiatry is comparable to that of Darwin in biology or Einstein in physics, coined the word 'schizophrenia' and classified the newly named disorder into various subtypes (hebephrenic, paranoid, catatonic). Significantly, Bleuler drew a clear distinction between what he thought were the primary disturbances in schizophrenia (autism and loosening of associations) and those he considered to be *secondary*, among which he included hallucinations and delusions. While Bleuler suspected that the primary disturbances might have a biological basis he was adamant that the secondary symptoms had a *psychological* origin. Indeed, he concluded that 'for the purpose of demonstrating clearly that the essence of the hallucinatory process lies in the psyche . . . no other disease is as well suited as schizophrenia.'[538] A consideration of the specific contents of the voices and delusions of people affected by schizophrenia convinced Bleuler that these symptoms developed on the basis of psychological processes:

> No one would hallucinate that Jesuits were persecuting him
> if he had never heard anything of the significance of Jesuits.
> The content of delusions and hallucinations can only be
> understood and conceived of in terms of definite external
> events. However, there can be no symptoms without
> content. Thus hallucinations and delusions . . . need not
> stem directly from the disease process itself. The latter
> provides only the predisposition, on the basis of which
> psychic processes develop the symptoms.[539]

Bleuler's views were strongly influenced by the psychodynamic perspective epitomised by Sigmund Freud and Carl Jung. In his own book on schizophrenia Jung noted that he and Bleuler fully agreed regarding the psychological origins of secondary symptoms:

I do not think it necessary to discuss in detail whether the secondary symptoms, as described by Bleuler, owe their existence and their specific form to psychological determination. Bleuler himself is fully convinced that their form and content, i.e. their individual phenomenology, are derived entirely from emotional complexes. I agree with Bleuler, whose experience of the psychogenesis of secondary symptoms coincides with my own, for we were collaborating in the years which preceded his famous book ... There can, indeed, be no doubt about the psychological determination of secondary symptoms.[540]

For a number of reasons the distinction between primary and secondary symptoms has been lost during the course of this century and it is now common for the *entire* symptomatology of schizophrenia to be attributed to putative biological causes. This major shift in thinking has had a number of significant consequences, not the least of which is the fact that little interest is now devoted to exploring the individualised thematic content of voices and delusions or to considering the possible purposes that these symptoms might serve in the overall context of the diagnosed person's life (these issues were discussed in Chapter Nine).

In spite of the vigorous efforts made in recent years to improve diagnostic reliability there is still probably no diagnosis in the whole of medicine about which there is more controversy than that of schizophrenia. Critics especially emphasise the limitations inherent in any approach which attempts to account for *every* aspect of schizophrenia (or any other functional mental disorder for that matter) in purely biological terms. In recent years a growing number of critical voices can be heard to emanate from within the ranks of the mental health professions. In an argument rather reminiscent of the views of Bleuler and Jung regarding the psychological origin of secondary symptoms the Irish psychiatrist David Healy has pointed out that voice experiences which occur in the context of functional mental disorders such as schizophrenia, depression and mania are far too complex to be adequately explained by the simplistic notion of a malfunctioning brain:

One strong indication that hallucinations result from fevers of the psyche rather than of the brain is that the perceptions involved are not just any perceptions as one might expect from abnormal brain function. Rather they are very specific perceptions ... Thus a depressed person will hear a voice abusing them, telling them they are worthless or damned, or urging them to kill themselves ... the hallucinations of mania and schizophrenia also reflect the concerns of affected subjects ... In contrast, organic brain disturbances – fevers of the brain, such as epilepsy, tumours, or drug or alcohol withdrawal – usually give rise to contentless or arbitrary perceptual phenomena, such as noises or flashes of light or colour rather than voices or visions ... A further pointer to the psychological nature of depressive or schizophrenic hallucinations comes from the experience of some normal people. It seems that some of us (10 percent) every so often have strikingly vivid visions on waking from sleep or on falling asleep. These are called hypnagogic hallucinations. The point that these hallucinations illustrate is that it is possible to have hallucinations when one's brain is functioning normally. Indeed to have detailed and complex hallucinations probably *requires* one's brain to be functioning normally ... Induction by hypnosis suggests that a prerequisite of complex hallucinations is an altered psychological state rather than an altered brain state.[541]

Some mental health professionals have gone further than simply calling for the adoption of a broader, more holistic approach and asked if it is useful to continue thinking of schizophrenia as an illness at all. In fact, a growing number of respected authorities have begun to suspect that, since many years of intensive research have failed to provide satisfactory answers to many of their most basic questions about this disturbance, the very notion that schizophrenia is an illness may actually be incorrect.[542] Some psychiatrists, including several who are internationally regarded authorities, have also begun asking whether it is useful to continue thinking of schizophrenia as an illness in the usual medical sense. One such person, Professor Luc Ciompi, believes that it is time to try a new approach. Professor Ciompi made the following statement in an article entitled 'Is There Really A Schizophrenia?', published in the *British Journal of Psychiatry* in 1984:

> It seems obvious that there is a schizophrenia, since our psychiatric institutions are filled with patients with this diagnosis ... Nevertheless, it is still doubtful whether the concept of a disease entity of schizophrenia is a correct one ... even Manfred Bleuler, the son of the author of the schizophrenia concept [Eugen Bleuler], has recently rejected this idea unequivocally. In fact, neither common causes nor satisfactory definitions of schizophrenia-like phenomena have emerged, and as our own long-term follow-up studies have shown, there is no uniform course. For these reasons, an alternative formulation should be tried.[543]

While these issues continue to stimulate heated debate a trend has emerged in sections of the mental health field which cuts through many of the complex conceptual and semantic issues concerning the validity of 'schizophrenia' and other psychiatric disorders. Adherents of this new approach have moved away from attempts to define, identify and treat supposed 'mental illnesses', choosing instead to focus on trying to understand how people develop individual symptoms (such as delusions and hallucinations) and how they can be helped if they are troubled by these particular experiences.[544] Instead of attributing a person's voice experiences to schizophrenia or some other 'psychotic illness' this pragmatic approach simply focuses on attempting to assist those who are troubled by voices or other phenomena. In distinct contrast to the commonplace practice of using non-specific methods such as neuroleptic drugs to treat the 'illness' as a whole, this approach is characterised by the use of *psychological* interventions which target a person's specific problems (e.g. disturbing voices or thoughts). Its potential advantages include the avoidance of a stigmatising diagnosis, the empowerment of people by teaching them practical techniques to use in coping with their problems, and the minimisation of problems with medication side-effects. (A broad range of psychological strategies for coping with disturbing voices were described in Chapter Eight.)

Encountering the Unexplained

The easiest way to deal with phenomena for which no ready explanation is available is to ignore them or declare them to be unreal. This has been done repeatedly throughout history by those who value certainty over truth. It has been common, for example, for people to simply dismiss various experiences involving the 'paranormal', or 'spirits', or any of the many other phenomena poorly accounted for by conventional Western belief systems, by conveniently labelling them as figments of the imagination or even as sensory deceptions. The cautious exercise of intelligent discernment is undoubtedly important when dealing with these kinds of experiences since it would be unwise to assume that *every* kind of sensory phenomenon is necessarily a true and accurate reflection of objective reality. Nevertheless, even when such discernment is applied there remain many sensory experiences which defy conventional explanation. In particular, some voice experiences entail qualities or characteristics which cannot be easily explained (or explained away!) by orthodox psychological or medical theories. Among these characteristics are the following:

• *Shared Perception*
Hearing voices is usually a purely personal and subjective experience. Voice experiences labelled as hallucinations are sometimes referred to as 'unshared' or 'private' perceptions to emphasise the fact that they are an inner experience (even though they may sometimes be perceived as coming from outside the hearer). While the majority of voice experiences *are* private there are some which appear to be shared with others. A classic example is the experience of Saul (St Paul) on the road to Damascus. According to the account provided in Acts (9:3–7) the men travelling with Saul also heard the voice of Jesus. The Bible contains numerous instances in which angels were perceived by groups of people and many examples of *collective* voice experiences (e.g. Matthew 17:1–8; John 12:27–30). In the latter instance the crowd standing by also heard the voice which spoke to Jesus who said of it, 'This voice has come for your sake, not for mine.' Students of parapsychology have recorded many examples in which a voice was heard by two or more people simultaneously. Thus, approximately 7% of the 493 voice

experiences reported in Professor Sidgwick's study were described as being collective; in some instances as many as five people claim to have heard the same voice.[545]

* *Correspondence with Objective Reality*

Voices sometimes appear to convey information regarding an external event which the hearer could not possibly have known about if it had not been for the voice experience. The so-called 'crisis apparitions' described in Chapter Six are an example of this phenomenon. Many instances have been reported in which a person has learnt about a remote event (such as an accident or the death of a loved one) as a result of hearing a voice, often that of the person involved in the event in question. (The term 'veridical' is sometimes used to indicate that a particular voice experience has corresponded with an actual outer event.)

* *Personhood and 'Otherness'*

While some voices are experienced as completely disembodied ('I just hear words hanging in the air') it is not uncommon for people to experience their voices as being intimately connected with one or a number of persons ('It is not just a voice I am hearing, it is a *person*'). Researchers have noted that some voices seem to have a well-developed 'personality' distinctly separate from that of the hearer. People who hear such voices sometimes give them names, attribute personal qualities to them (e.g. friendliness, kindness, moodiness, spitefulness), and some even describe their physical appearance. Some people develop complex and multi-faceted interpersonal 'relationships' with such voices, which may even involve a sexual aspect.

* *Physical Influence and Control*

The experiences some people have with voices go beyond simply hearing them. Researchers have found that voices are sometimes reported to have the ability to induce physical sensations, inflict pain, or even control parts of the hearer's body. Professor Eugen Bleuler noted that 'The voices not only speak to the patient, but they pass electricity through his body, beat him, paralyse him, take his thoughts away.'[546] The so-called 'Lower Order' voices described by Wilson Van Dusen often threatened pain as a way of reinforcing their power and were apparently able to produce physical pain indistinguishable from ordinary pain, the only difference being that the voices would threaten it just before it was felt. Some people have described participating in sexual activities with their voices and experiencing sexual gratification as a result.[547]

• *Knowledge and Wisdom*

Voices sometimes provide people with knowledge or information they did not previously possess. Many creative individuals have been inspired by voices and in some instances have even had work 'dictated' to them. Many people have received spiritual guidance by way of voice experiences. In some instances their lives have influenced the course of human history (e.g. Joan of Arc). Some saints who reached the acme of spiritual understanding were guided and instructed by voices. As described in Chapter Two, works allegedly produced by practitioners of 'trance channelling' occasionally demonstrate a high level of sophistication. Some mediums are apparently able to gain access to information about deceased individuals as a result of their ability to converse with 'spirit voices'. So-called 'Higher Order' voices have been known to demonstrate a profound knowledge of subjects about which the hearer was entirely ignorant; they may even employ a vocabulary and use technical terms and concepts well beyond the hearer's level of education or prior knowledge. Jung credited his 'guiding spirit', Philemon, with knowledge and wisdom vastly superior to his own.

• *Malevolence*

Some voice experiences are characterised by an extreme degree of malevolence. In such cases the hearer may be assailed by several (and often by many) hostile, critical or viciously attacking voices having an apparently malevolent intent. Such voices may be strikingly perverse, urging or even ordering a particular action and then criticising the person for carrying it out. Ordinarily gentle persons sometimes experience prolonged harangues by voices incessantly urging them to commit uncharacteristic acts, possibly even violence. So-called 'Lower Order' voices are often vehemently anti-religious and will mock any attempt by the hearer to engage in religious practices.

• *Persistence*

Voices which occur in the context of mental disorder are sometimes remarkably persistent despite intensive therapeutic interventions. For example, people who begin hearing voices during an acute psychotic episode sometimes continue to hear them long after the psychosis has abated. Some persons living with schizophrenia continue to hear voices over prolonged periods, possibly even for many years (although often at a diminished level of intensity), in spite of their compliance with prescribed medication regimens. (Such persons are sometimes described as 'treatment resistant', although other symptoms such as delusions and thought disorder may have been significantly ameliorated by the drugs.)

The existence of these and possibly other enigmatic characteristics underscores the fact that hearing voices is not a unitary phenomenon for which a single, simple explanation is likely to be found. The truth is that, while the various theories outlined in Chapter Six undoubtedly contribute toward our understanding of how and why voices occur, our ability to explain these experiences remains extremely limited. It is likely that in order to achieve a better understanding of voices and related phenomena we will need to expand our view of reality and acknowledge the existence of realms of experience beyond those familiar to our everyday consciousness. William James recognised this need at the beginning of the twentieth century. Having spent many years studying and reflecting upon the varieties of human experience he concluded:

> Our normal waking consciousness, rational consciousness as we call it, is but one special type of consciousness, whilst all about it, parted from it by the filmiest of screens, there lie potential forms of consciousness entirely different. We may go through life without suspecting their existence; but apply the requisite stimulus, and at a touch they are there in all their completeness, definite types of mentality which probably somewhere have their field of application and adaptation. No account of the universe in its totality can be final which leaves these other forms of consciousness quite disregarded. How to regard them is the question – for they are so discontinuous with ordinary consciousness. Yet they may determine attitudes though they cannot furnish formulas, and open a region though they fail to give a map. At any rate, they forbid a premature closing of our accounts with reality.[548]

Returning the Psyche to the Centre

As the new millenium begins we might well look in wonderment at the extraordinary range of scientific and technological discoveries that have been made in recent years and the rate at which our understanding of the physical world is increasing. Officially declared the 'Decade of the Brain', the 1990s in particular have seen an unprecedented accumulation of knowledge regarding the structure and function of the organ which is arguably the acme of human biological evolution. This new information is enormously important and holds the promise of important advances in a number of areas. It is quite likely, for example, that within the next few years significant progress will be made toward unravelling the complex mechanisms associated with hallucinatory perception and the neurological correlates of certain mental disorders.

While research accelerates in the physical domain many people now experience a deep hunger for something other than more technical information. In the early 1900s Carl Jung warned of the limitations of a one-sidedly materalistic approach to human behaviour and suggested that trying to understand the workings of the mind by studying the brain alone was like attempting to decipher the meaning and purpose of a structure such as a cathedral by conducting a mineralogical analysis of the stones used in its construction. Increasingly, Jung's intuitions appear to have been correct. Thus, when the world-renowned neurosurgeon and researcher Wilder Penfield reviewed his life's work in his book, *The Mystery of the Mind*, he declared his disbelief that consciousness is a product of the workings of the brain or that it will ever be accounted for solely in terms of cerebral anatomy and physiology.[549]

A thoughtful consideration of the vast range of experiences which in one way or another involve hearing voices underscores William James's observation that the apparently solid physical world of ordinary waking consciousness (which is often equated with 'reality') is but one among many possible worlds of experience. Others also exist – including the dream world, the spirit world, the world of the imagination – and give rise to experiences which immeasurably enrich the texture of our lives. While the various worlds generally remain discrete they may at certain times become continuous, thus allowing images and experiences to filter into our awareness from beyond the boundaries of the everyday and physical. Whether these 'other worlds' are entirely subjective or if they may yet prove to have aspects which correspond to some degree with objective reality is a question which will doubtless occupy the talents of researchers for many years to come.

To remain open to the existence of these other realms, or even to simply think about them in an open-minded way, requires considerable courage for they challenge not only our usual beliefs about the nature of reality but also our very sense of self-identity. And yet, as the German poet Rainer Maria Rilke felt, it may be that it is only those who are 'ready for anything, who exclude nothing' who truly live in the fullness of their own being and of life itself:

> We must assume our existence as *broadly* as we in any way can; everything, even the unheard-of, must be possible in it. That is at bottom the only courage that is demanded of us: to have the courage for the most strange, the most singular and the most inexplicable that we may encounter. That mankind has in this sense been cowardly has done life endless harm; the experiences that are called 'visions', the whole so-called 'spirit-world', death, all those things that are so closely akin to us, have by daily parrying been so crowded out of life that the senses with which we could have grasped them are atrophied. To say nothing of God. But fear of the inexplicable has not alone impoverished the existence of the individual; the relationship between one human being and another has also been cramped by it, as though it had been lifted out of the riverbed of endless possibilities and set down in a fallow spot on the bank, to which nothing happens ... only someone who is ready for everything, who excludes nothing, not even the most enigmatical, will live the relation to another as something alive and will himself draw exhaustively from his own existence.[550]

What is needed now, above all, is a new approach which places the psyche – the human soul or spirit – at the *centre* of our considerations rather than dismissing it as an illusion or a mere epiphenomenon of brain functioning. After all, life would not even exist for human beings were it not for the fact that it is reflected in the psyche. Such a world-view would allow the integration of living human experience and objective scientific research to create an holistic perspective which recognises and values the importance of *all* aspects of life. In the end, the development of such a view may depend on our willingness to re-evaluate our usual way of perceiving ourselves and the extraordinary world we live in.

RECOMMENDED READING

Consciousness/Transpersonal Psychology/Parapsychology

* *Inner Voice Experiences: An Exploratory Study of Thirty Cases* by Myrtle Heery (*Journal of Transpersonal Psychology*, Vol.21, No.1, 1989.)
* *Inner Voices: Distinguishing Transcendent and Pathological Characteristics* by Mitchell Liester (*Journal of Transpersonal Psychology*, Vol.28, No.1, 1996)
* *Beyond the Brain* by Stanislav Grof (New York: State University of New York Press, 1985)
* *The Cosmic Game* by Stanislav Grof (Hill of Content Publishing, 1998)
* *The Origin of Consciousness in the Breakdown of the Bicameral Mind* by Julian Jaynes (Boston: Houghton Mifflin, 1982)
* *Exploring the Paranormal: Perspectives on Belief and Experience* by George Zollschan, John Schumaker and Greg Walsh (eds) (Lindfield, NSW: Unity Press, 1989)

Jungian and Post-Jungian Psychology

* *Memories, Dreams, Reflections* by C.G.Jung (London: Fontana, 1967)
* *Re-Visioning Psychology* by James Hillman (New York: Harper and Row, 1977)
* *Boundaries of the Soul: The Practice of Jung's Psychology* by June Singer (New York: Anchor Books, 1973)
* *Invisible Guests: The Development of Imaginal Dialogues* by Mary Watkins (Boston: Sigo Press, 1990)

Spirituality/Inner World

* *The Varieties of Religious Experience* by William James (Penguin, 1982)
* *The Natural Depth in Man* by Wilson Van Dusen (New York: Swedenborg Foundation, 1972)
* *The Interior Castle* by Teresa of Avila (New York: Paulist Press, 1979)

- *The Exploration of the Inner World* by Anton Boisen (Philadelphia: University of Philadelphia Press, 1971)

Personal Growth

- *Discover Your Subpersonalities* by John Rowan (London: Routledge, 1993)
- *Inner Work: Using Dreams and Active Imagination for Personal Growth* by Robert Johnson (San Francisco: Harper and Row, 1989)
- *The Stormy Search for the Self: A Guide to Personal Growth Through Transformational Crisis* by Christina Grof and Stanislav Grof (Los Angeles: Jeremy Tarcher, 1990)
- *Embracing Our Selves* by Hal Stone and Sidra Winkleman (SanRafael, California: New World Library, 1989)

Near Death Experience

- *Life after Life* by Raymond Moody (Atlanta, GA: Mockingbird Books, 1975)
- *Within the Light* by Cherie Sutherland (Sydney: Bantam Books, 1993)

Shamanism

- *Shamanism: Archaic Technique of Ecstasy* by Mercia Eliade (London: Arkana, 1989)
- *The Spirit of Shamanism* by Roger Walsh (London: Harper-Collins, 1990)
- *Dreamtime and Inner Space: The World of the Shaman* by Holger Kalweit (Boston: Shambala, 1988)

Holistic Approaches to Schizophrenia/Voices

- *Understanding and Helping the Schizophrenic* by Silvano Arieti (Penguin Books, 1981)
- *Healing the Split* by John Nelson (Los Angeles: Jeremy Tarcher, 1990)
- *Living With Schizophrenia* by John Watkins (Melbourne: Hill Of Content, 1996)
- *Hearing Voices: A Self-Help Guide and Reference Book* by John Watkins (Melbourne: Richmond Fellowship of Victoria, 1993)

APPENDIX
RESOURCES AND SUPPORT

HEARING VOICES NETWORK

Originating in the Netherlands in the late 1980s, this self-help movement has grown into a world-wide network whose aim is to provide information and support to people who hear voices, their relatives and carers, and mental health workers. Activities auspiced by the various members of the network include regional support groups, education and training, newsletters, online forums, and telephone help-lines.

Australia

The Hearing Voices Network Australia (HVNA) is auspiced by Richmond Fellowship of Western Australia. www.rfwa.org.au

United Kingdom

The UK Hearing Voices Network celebrated its 15th anniversary in 2006, at which time there were nearly two hundred affiliated support groups throughout the United Kingdom. www.hearing-voices.org

United States of America

This network is co-ordinating the development and activities of support groups, education, and training for voice hearers and their allies throughout the USA. www.hvn-usa.org

INTERVOICE

INTERVOICE is the International Network of Training, Education and Research into Hearing Voices. The activities of this international online community include education and training, an annual conference, and hosting interactive online forums. On September 14th, 2006 INTERVOICE auspiced the first 'World Hearing Voices Day', now an annual event with events and activities in many different countries. www.intervoiceonline.org

TRAUMA AND DISSOCIATION

The International Society for the Study of Trauma and Dissociation: primarily for mental health professionals, the ISSTD is a non-profit association whose purpose is to develop and promote effective clinical responses to problems related to trauma and dissociation via training, conferences, and the *Journal of Trauma and Dissociation*. www.isst-d.org

Dissociation Australia: This group provides Australian professionals, students, and public with reliable, up-to-date information about dissociation and dissociative disorders. www.arts.monash.edu.au/behaviour/dissociation

288

NOTES

Chapter One
1 Liester, 1996, p.26.
2 Sidgwick et al., 1894.
3 West, 1948; Forrer, 1960; Pitts et al., 1961; Mott et al., 1965; McKellar, 1968; Bentall and Slade, 1985; Young et al., 1986.
4 Posey and Losch, 1983, p.107.
5 Heery, 1989.
6 Tien, 1991.
7 Barrett and Etheridge, 1992.
8 Jaynes, 1986, p.526.
9 Esquirol, 1965, p.110.
10 Galton, 1973, p.121.
11 James, 1948, p.331.
12 Mavromatis, 1987, p.34.
13 Van Dusen, 1972, p.86.
14 Tyrrell, 1953; Mavromatis, 1987.
15 Stevenson, 1983.
16 Kaplan and Sadock, 1981.
17 Bleuler, 1950, p.440.
18 Bilu and Abramovitch, 1985.
19 Singer, 1973a.
20 Jaynes, 1986, p.527.
21 Grimby, 1993.
22 Posey and Losch, 1983, p.110.
23 Rees, 1971.
24 Kaplan and Sadock, 1989.
25 Matchett, 1972.
26 Olson et al., 1985.
27 Jaynes, 1982, p.86.
28 Smith, 1997.
29 Yamamoto et al., 1969.
30 Al-Issa, 1978.
31 Slade and Bentall, 1988; Grassian, 1983; Siegel, 1984.
32 Wilcox et al., 1991.
33 Hay, 1982, p.139.
34 Forrer, 1960, p.95.
35 Ensink, 1992.
36 Bliss, 1980; Ross, 1989.
37 Brauschi and West, 1959; Asaad and Shapiro, 1986; Slade and Bentall, 1988.
38 Lilly, 1956; Leff, 1968; Zuckerman, 1969.
39 Storr, 1989.
40 Kaplan and Sadock, 1981, p.116.
41 Lilly, 1956; Slade and Bentall, 1988.
42 Lindbergh, 1953, pp.389–390.
43 Hamilton, 1985.
44 Asaad and Shapiro, 1986; Hammeke et al. 1983; Keshavan et al., 1992.
45 Slade and Bentall, 1988.
46 Meier, 1989.
47 Slade and Bentall, 1988.
48 Erickson, 1969, p.63.
49 Bliss et al., 1983.
50 Moody, 1975; Greyson and Stevenson, 1980.
51 Sabom, 1982.
52 Sutherland, 1993.
53 Sutherland, 1993, p.131.
54 Sutherland, 1993, p.210.
55 Sutherland, 1993, p.295.
56 Grof, 1985.
57 Masters and Houston, 1966, p.14.
58 Harner, 1973, p.102.
59 Jaynes, 1982.
60 Underhill, 1990.
61 Porter, 1989, p.67.
62 Milner, 1978, p.48.
63 Storr, 1983, p.199.
64 Chatterjee, 1984.
65 de Beauvoir, 1963, p.181.
66 Peck, 1985, p.136.
67 Lukoff, 1990.
68 Slade and Bentall, 1988.
69 Allen and Agus, 1968.
70 Slade and Bentall, 1988.

71 Asaad and Shapiro, 1986; Slade and Bentall, 1988.
72 Kaplan and Sadock, 1981.
73 Goetz et al., 1982; Sacks, 1991.
74 Jaynes, 1982; Heery, 1989; Liester, 1996.
75 Freud, 1966, p.261.
76 Cross, 1914, p.250.
77 Jung, 1967, p.207.

Chapter Two
78 Cited in Liester, 1996, p.25.
79 Underhill, 1990, p.269.
80 Heery, 1989, p.75.
81 Jaynes, 1982, p.323.
82 James, 1902, p.467.
83 Kroll and Bachrach, 1982a; Kroll and Bachrach, 1982b.
84 Underhill, 1990, p.268.
85 Teresa of Avila, 1979, p.119–120.
86 Underhill, 1990, p.273.
87 Gurney et al., 1970, p.480.
88 St John of the Cross, 1964, p.132.
89 Aumann, 1967, p.953.
90 Underhill, 1990, p.181.
91 Underhill, 1990, p.276.
92 Cristiani, 1977.
93 Cited in Liester, 1996, p.12.
94 Underhill, 1990, p.278.
95 Thomas à Kempis, 1963, p.176.
96 James, 1902, p.468.
97 St Teresa, 1979, p.123.
98 James, 1902, p.328.
99 Talmage, 1970, p.760.
100 Starbuck, 1899, p.78.
101 Hardy, 1979, p.40.
102 McKenna and Libersat, 1987, p.5.
103 Connell, 1992.
104 Bucke, 1961, p.105.
105 Hardy, 1979.
106 Hardy, 1979, p.40.
107 Posey and Losch, 1983.
108 Romme and Escher, 1989.
109 Heery, 1989.
110 Heery, 1989, p.75.
111 Jaynes, 1986.
112 Craciunas, 1961.
113 Cited in Honig, 1973, p.74.

114 Swedenborg, 1971, p.136.
115 Jung, 1977, p.26.
116 Guirdham, 1982.
117 Cited in Kalweit, 1988, p.vii.
118 Grof and Grof, 1990, p.93.
119 Foundation For Inner Peace, 1985.
120 Elkin, 1977; Eliade, 1989; Walsh, 1990.
121 Eliade, 1989.
122 Neihardt, 1988, p.41.
123 Neihardt, 1988, p.49.
124 Eliade, 1989, p.39.
125 Bourguignon, 1970.
126 Eshowsky, 1993.

Chapter Three
127 Bleuler, 1950, p.351.
128 Al-Issa, 1978.
129 Kroll and Bachrach, 1982a.
130 Sarbin and Juhasz, 1967.
131 Esquirol, 1965, p.93.
132 American Psychiatric Association, 1994, p.767.
133 Hall, Popkin and Faillace, 1978.
134 Kulkarni, Copolov, and Keks, 1991.
135 Kaplan and Sadock, 1981.
136 Mayer-Gross et al., 1960.
137 American Psychiatric Association, 1987.
138 Kaplan and Sadock, 1981.
139 Alpert and Silvers, 1970.
140 Mayer-Gross et al., 1960, p.358.
141 Kaplan and Sadock, 1981.
142 Schatzberg and Rothschild, 1992.
143 Taylor and Abrams, 1975.
144 Wing, 1978.
145 Carlson and Goodwin, 1973.
146 American Psychiatric Association, 1994.
147 Sartorius et al., 1974.
148 American Psychiatric Association, 1994, p.767.
149 American Psychiatric Association, 1987.
150 Ross, 1989.
151 Nelson, 1990, p.209.
152 Bliss, 1980.

153 Ross et al., 1990.
154 Ross, 1989, p.100.
155 American Psychiatric Association, 1994.
156 Ensink, 1992.
157 Mueser and Butler, 1987; Wilcox et al., 1991.
158 Mueser and Butler, 1987, p.301.
159 McGorry et al., 1991.
160 Kaplan and Sadock, 1981.
161 Farley et al., 1968.
162 Levinson, 1966; Sirota et al., 1987.
163 Andrade and Srinath, 1986, p.101.
164 Rack, 1982.
165 Romme and Escher, 1996.
166 Modell, 1960.
167 Arieti, 1981.

Chapter Four
168 Bleuler, 1950, p.388.
169 Slade and Bentall, 1988; Boyle, 1993; Thomas, 1997.
170 Rosenhan, 1973.
171 Hamilton, 1976, p.47.
172 Bleuler, 1950, p.96.
173 Jaynes, 1982, p.88.
174 Bateson, 1961, p.117.
175 Bleuler, 1950, p.116.
176 Farr, 1982, p.2.
177 Nelson, 1990, p.207.
178 Vonnegut, 1976, p.136.
179 King, 1956, cited in Kaplan, 1964, p.134.
180 Bleuler, 1950, p.387.
181 Benjamin, 1989; Romme and Escher, 1989.
182 Bateson, 1961, p.285.
183 Schreber, 1955, cited in Torrey, 1988, p.49.
184 Bleuler, 1950.
185 Bleuler, 1950, p.113.
186 Jaynes, 1982, p.95.
187 North, 1989, p.26.
188 Farr, 1982, p.6.
189 Alpert and Silvers, 1970; Romme and Escher, 1996.

190 Farr, 1982, p.2.
191 Jaynes, 1982.
192 Bleuler, 1950.
193 Jaspers, 1963, p.73.
194 Bleuler, 1950, p.99.
195 Bleuler, 1950, p.110.
196 Sechehaye, 1970, p.42.
197 Romme et al., 1992.
198 Van Dusen, 1972, p.140.
199 Bleuler, 1950, p.97.
200 Aggernaes, 1972.
201 Chadwick and Birchwood, 1994.
202 King, 1956, cited in Kaplan, 1964, p.135.
203 Bleuler, 1950.
204 American Psychiatric Association, 1994.
205 Bleuler, 1950.
206 Jung, 1974.
207 Schreber, 1955, cited in Peterson, 1982, p.155.
208 Bleuler, 1950, p.96.
209 Jaspers, 1963; Watkins, 1990.
210 Bleuler, 1950, p.97.
211 Farr, 1982, p.2.
212 Jaspers, 1963, p.73.
213 American Psychiatric Association, 1994.
214 Folkard, 1992, p.86.
215 MacDonald, 1960, p.175.
216 Hellerstein et al., 1987.
217 Junginger, 1990.
218 Farr, 1982, p.4.
219 Bateson, 1961, p.277.
220 Mott et al., 1965.
221 Judkins and Slade, 1981.
222 Benjamin, 1989, p.307.
223 Modell, 1960.
224 Boisen, 1960, cited in Kaplan, 1964, p.121.
225 Bleuler, 1950, p.104.
226 Bateson, 1961, p.69.
227 Falloon and Talbot, 1981; Romme and Escher, 1989.
228 Nelson, 1990, p.213.
229 Falloon and Talbot, 1981; Carr, 1988; Benjamin, 1989.

230 Leete, 1993, cited in Hatfield and Lefley, 1993, p.117.
231 Folkard, 1992, p.19.
232 Romme and Escher, 1989, p.210.
233 King, 1956, in Kaplan, 1964, p.134.
234 Folkard, 1992, p.21.
235 Farr, 1982, p.1.
236 Folkard, 1992, p.22.
237 Rollin, 1980, p.146.
238 Lally, 1989.
239 Lally, 1989, p.260.
240 Rollin, 1980, p.150.
241 Cromwell and Snyder, 1993.
242 Sechehaye, 1970, p.80.
243 Folkard, 1992, p.127.
244 Romme et al., 1992.
245 Watkins, 1996.
246 Falloon, 1987, p.181.
247 Folkard, 1992, pp.24–25.
248 North, 1989, p.139.
249 Anonymous, 1997, p.11.
250 Larkin, 1979.
251 Vonnegut, 1976, p.137.
252 Falloon and Talbot, 1981; Romme and Escher, 1989.
253 Modell, 1960; Benjamin, 1989.
254 Arieti, 1981; Benjamin, 1989.
255 Modell, 1960; Lockhart, 1975.
256 Lewinsohn, 1968.
257 Brier and Strauss, 1983; Falloon, 1987; Carr, 1988.

Chapter Five
258 Jaspers, 1963, p.128–130.
259 American Psychiatric Association, 1994.
260 Thigpen and Cleckley, 1957.
261 Schreiber, 1973.
262 Casey and Wilson, 1993.
263 Coté, 1994.
264 Ross, 1989.
265 American Psychiatric Association, 1994.
266 Ross, 1989, p.72.
267 Benjamin, 1989, p.306.
268 Bliss, 1980, p.1389.

269 Richards, 1990; APA, 1994; Nelson, 1990.
270 Densen-Gerber, 1986.
271 Bliss et al., 1983, p.31.
272 Ross, 1989; Coté, 1994.
273 Ross, 1989.
274 Sizemore and Pittillo, 1978, p.254.
275 Ross, 1989.
276 Bliss, 1980.
277 Bliss, 1980, p.1394.
278 Noll, 1989, p.365.
279 Ross, 1989.
280 Ross, 1989, p.115.
281 Ross, 1989.
282 Ross, 1989; Boon and Draijer, 1993.
283 Ross, 1989.
284 Ross et al., 1990.
285 Bliss et al., 1983.
286 Rosenbaum, 1980.
287 Ross, 1989.
288 Ross, 1989, p.162.
289 Ross 1989, p.101.
290 Bliss et al., 1983.
291 Ross, 1989, p.163.
292 Bliss et al., 1983.
293 Ross, 1989, p.192.
294 Richards, 1990.
295 Boon and Draijer, 1993.
296 Torrey, 1988, p.109.
297 Rosenbaum, 1980, p.1384.
298 Bleuler, 1979, p.1404.
299 Healy, 1990.
300 Beck and van der Kolk, 1987; Bryer et al., 1987.
301 Walsh, 1990, p.128.

Chapter Six
302 Liester, 1996, p.25.
303 Strauss, 1969.
304 Benjamin, 1989, p.306.
305 Green and Kinsbourne, 1990.
306 Gould, 1950, cited in Smith, 1992, p.170.
307 Shaw, 1957, p.9.
308 Cited in Watkins, 1990, p.98.
309 Stephen, 1989, p.61.

310 Levinson, 1966, p.20, emphasis in original.
311 Jung, 1974, p.148.
312 Reil, 1803, cited in Ellenberger, 1970, p.147.
313 Berne, 1975, p.273.
314 Australian Broadcasting Commission, 1984.
315 Modell, 1960.
316 Arieti, 1981.
317 Jung, 1937, cited in Noll, 1989, p.356.
318 Jung, 1977, p.138, emphasis in original.
319 Richards, 1990.
320 Ferrucci, 1982, p.48.
321 Assagioli, 1975.
322 Berne, 1975.
323 Stone and Winkelman, 1989.
324 Stone and Winkelman, 1989, p.50.
325 Stone and Winkelman, 1989, p.60.
326 Singer, 1973b, p.95.
327 Jung, 1969, p.115.
328 Perry, 1989.
329 Jung, 1967, p.207.
330 James, 1986.
331 Nelson, 1989.
332 Gurney et al., 1970. (Vol.1, p.482)
333 Tyrrell, 1953.
334 Malinak et al., 1979, p.1154.
335 Stevenson, 1983, p.1609.
336 Sandford and Sandford, 1985, p.318.
337 Greyson, 1977.
338 Ross, 1989.
339 Ehrenwald, 1978.
340 Nelson, 1990, p.324.
341 Dean et al., 1980.
342 Freud, 1966, p.261.
343 Devereux, 1970.
344 Clark, 1980, p.276.
345 Heery, 1989; Liester, 1996.
346 Lukoff, 1985.
347 Grof and Grof, 1990.
348 Bragdon, 1990, p.125.

349 Chadwick and Birchwood, 1994.
350 Tart cited in Walsh, 1990, p.132.
351 Bliss et al., 1983, p.32.
352 Bliss, 1980.
353 Bliss et al., 1983.
354 Jaynes, 1982, p.397.
355 Jaynes, 1982.
356 Jaynes, 1982, p.93.
357 Jaynes, 1982, p.405.
358 Slade, 1976; Hoffman, 1986.
359 Frith, 1979.
360 MacDonald, 1960, p.175.
361 Slade and Bentall, 1988.
362 Torrey, 1988, p.50.
363 Cleghorn et al., 1992; Tiihonen et al., 1992.
364 Gabbard, 1992.
365 Bleuler, 1950; Modell, 1960; Jung, 1974; Arieti, 1981.
366 Asaad and Shapiro, 1986, p.1095.
367 Bentall, 1990; Boyle, 1993; Thomas, 1997.
368 Romme and Escher, 1989.

Chapter Seven
369 Fox and Sheldrake, 1996, p.xii.
370 Kelsey, 1978.
371 Kelsey, 1978, p.53
372 Fox and Sheldrake, 1996.
373 Slocum, 1978, p.59.
374 Osis, 1961; Osis and Haraldsson, 1977; Barrett, 1986.
375 Bourguignon, 1970.
376 Kalweit, 1988, p.122.
377 Lukoff, 1990, p.27.
378 Grof and Grof, 1990.
379 Lukoff, 1990, p.24.
380 Lukoff, 1990, p.26.
381 Brown, 1971.
382 Brown, 1975.
383 Stokes and Dearsley, 1980.
384 Ross, 1989.
385 Jung, 1977, p.111.
386 King, 1956, in Kaplan, 1964, p.135.
387 Warner, 1985.
388 Van Dusen, 1972.
389 Van Dusen, 1973, p.122.

390 Whitwell and Barker, 1980.
391 Nelson, 1990.
392 Van Dusen, 1972, p.144.
393 Van Dusen, 1973, p.133.
394 Van Dusen, 1973, p.124.
395 Cited in Kalweit, 1988, p.111.
396 Jung, 1973, cited in Noll, 1987, p.60.
397 Julian, 1987.
398 Chadwick and Birchwood, 1994.
399 Van Dusen, 1972, p.148.
400 Kroll and Bachrach, 1982a.
401 King, 1956, in Kaplan, 1964, p.135
402 Al-Issa, 1978; Eliade,1989.
403 Cited in Van Dusen, 1972, p.136.
404 St John of the Cross, 1964, pp.204–206.
405 Clifford, 1989, p.151.
406 Chadwick and Birchwood, 1994.
407 Bateson, 1961, p.271.
408 St John of the Cross, 1964, p.132.
409 St John of the Cross, 1964, p.202.
410 St John of the Cross, 1964, p.133.
411 St John of the Cross, 1964, p.209.
412 St Teresa of Avila, 1979, p.125.
413 St Teresa of Avila, 1979, p.125.
414 St John of the Cross, 1964, p.133.
415 Fox and Sheldrake, 1996.
416 Schreber, 1955.
417 Schreber, 1955, cited in Kaplan, 1964, p.131.

Chapter Eight
418 Lovejoy, 1984, p.812.
419 Corday, 1989, p.74.
420 Al-Issa, 1978.
421 Warner, 1985, p.162.
422 Stevenson, 1983, p.1609.
423 Slade, 1976.
424 Allen and Agus, 1968.
425 Handel, 1987.
426 Bateson, 1961, p.294.
427 Arieti, 1980, p.468, emphasis in original.
428 Podvoll, 1990, p.46.
429 Slade and Bentall, 1988.
430 Lovejoy, 1984, p.811.

431 MacDonald, 1960, p.180.
432 Goff et al., 1992.
433 Rollin, 1980, p.124.
434 Brier and Strauss, 1983; Kanas and Barr, 1984; Falloon, 1987; Tarrier, 1992.
435 Falloon and Talbot, 1981.
436 Green and Kinsbourne, 1990; Nelson et al., 1991.
437 Handel, 1987.
438 Rollin, 1980, p.147.
439 Falloon and Talbot, 1981.
440 Carr, 1988.
441 Nelson et al., 1991.
442 Collins et al., 1989.
443 Feder, 1982; Collins et al., 1989; Nelson et al., 1991.
444 Margo et al., 1981.
445 McInnis and Marks, 1990.
446 Carr, 1988, p.349.
447 Handel, 1987.
448 Field, 1985.
449 Weingaertner, 1971.
450 Falloon and Talbot, 1981.
451 Slade and Bentall, 1988.
452 Australian Broadcasting Commission, 1984.
453 Romme et al., 1992, p.102.
454 Chadwick and Birchwood, 1994.
455 Greene, 1978.
456 Romme and Escher, 1989, p.212.
457 Lovejoy, 1984, p.811.
458 Handel, 1987.
459 Weingaertner, 1971.
460 Romme and Escher, 1989, p.209.
461 Strauss, 1989.
462 Torrey, 1988.
463 Carr, 1983; Tarrier, 1992.
464 Healy, 1993.
465 Kaplan and Sadock, 1981, p.252.
466 Watkins, 1996.
467 Healy, 1989.
468 Beckman and Haas, 1980; Lingjaerde, 1982.
469 Falloon and Talbot, 1981.

Chapter Nine
470 Hillman and Ventura, 1992, p.10.
471 Gabbard, 1992.
472 Will, 1962, p.180.
473 Sacks, 1991, p.215.
474 Sacks, 1991, p.169, emphasis added.
475 Sacks, 1991, p.170.
476 Miller et al., 1993.
477 Maitland, 1997, p.10.
478 Modell, 1960, p.64.
479 Benjamin, 1989.
480 Larkin, 1979.
481 Boss, 1963; Lockhart, 1975; Falloon and Talbot, 1981; Romme and Escher, 1989.
482 Slade and Bentall, 1988.
483 Haddock et al., 1996.
484 Thomas, 1997, p.186.
485 Strauss, 1989, p.182.
486 Handel, 1987.
487 Slade and Bentall, 1988.
488 Handel, 1987.
489 Kingdon and Turkington, 1991.
490 Handel, 1987.
491 Corday, 1989, p.74.
492 Bleuler, 1950, p.485.
493 Bleuler, 1950, p.388.
494 Jung, 1974, p.90.
495 Eigen, 1993, p.47.
496 Bleuler, 1950, pp.96–97.
497 Boisen, 1971, p.56.
498 Macnab, 1966, p.21.
499 Handel, 1987.
500 Handel, 1987.
501 Bateson, 1961, p.270.
502 Rojcewicz and Rojcewicz, 1997.
503 Handel, 1987.
504 Romme and Escher, 1989, p.211.
505 Podvoll, 1990, p.246.
506 Handel, 1987.
507 Watkins, 1990.
508 Ross, 1989, p.115.
509 Rilke, 1954, p.69.
510 Ribi, 1990, p.29.
511 Handel, 1987.
512 Richards, 1990.

513 Jung, 1967, p.148.
514 Van Dusen, 1973, p.132.
515 Johnson, 1989, p.138.
516 Johnson, 1989, p.139.
517 Lockhart, 1975, p.149.
518 Lockhart, 1975, p.149.
519 Lockhart, 1975, p.151.
520 Lockhart, 1975, p.158.
521 Sanford, 1977, p.143.
522 Jung, 1967, p.214.

Epilogue
523 Jung, 1969, p.79.
524 Romme and Escher, 1989, p.210.
525 Romme and Escher, 1989, p.215.
526 American Psychiatric Association, 1994, p.767.
527 Galton, 1973, p.127.
528 Forrer, 1960.
529 Stevenson, 1983.
530 Tyrrell, 1953, p.24.
531 Ross, 1989, p.183.
532 Grof, 1985; Lukoff, 1985; Nelson, 1990; Podvoll, 1990.
533 Jung, 1977, p.125.
534 Grof, 1985.
535 Boyle, 1993; Thomas, 1997.
536 Brigitte, Sue, Mem and Veronika, 1996, p.11.
537 Brigitte, Sue, Mem and Veronika, 1996, p.11.
538 Bleuler, 1950, p.388.
539 Bleuler, 1950, p.349.
540 Jung, 1974, p.158.
541 Healy, 1990, pp.163–165, emphasis added.
542 Bentall et al., 1988; Bentall, 1990; Boyle, 1993.
543 Ciompi, 1984, p.636.
544 Slade and Bentall, 1988; Slade, 1990; Tarrier, 1992; Haddock and Slade, 1996.
545 Tyrrell, 1953.
546 Bleuler, 1950, p.97.
547 Modell, 1960; Van Dusen, 1972.
548 James, 1902, p.378.
549 Penfield, 1976.
550 Rilke, 1954, p.67.

REFERENCES

Aggernaes,A. (1972) The Experienced Reality of Hallucinations and Other Psychological Phenomena, *Acta Psychiatrica Scandinavica*, Vol.48.

Al-Issa,I. (1978) Sociocultural Factors in Hallucinations. *International Journal of Social Psychiatry*, Vol.24, No.1.

Allen,T. and Agus,B. (1968) Hyperventilation Leading to Hallucinations. *American Journal of Psychiatry*, 125:5.

Alpert,M. and Silvers,K. (1970) Perceptual Characteristics Distinguishing Auditory Hallucinations in Schizophrenia and Acute Alcoholic Psychoses. *American Journal of Psychiatry*, 127:3.

American Psychiatric Association (1987) *Diagnostic and Statistical Manual of Mental Disorders – Third Edition – Revised* (DSM-III-R). Washington, DC, American Psychiatric Association.

American Psychiatric Association (1994) *Diagnostic and Statistical Manual of Mental Disorders – Fourth Edition (DSM-IV)*. Washington, DC, American Psychiatric Association.

Andrade,C. and Srinath,S. (1986) True Auditory Hallucinations as a Conversion Symptom. *British Journal of Psychiatry*, Vol.148.

Anonymous (1997) Companions on a Journey: An Exploration of an Alternative Community Mental Health Project. *Dulwich Centre Newsletter*, No.1.

Arieti,S. (1980) Psychotherapy of Schizophrenia: New or Revised Procedures. *American Journal of Psychotherapy*, Vol.XXXIV, No.4.

Arieti,S. (1981) *Understanding and Helping the Schizophrenic: A Guide for Family and Friends.* Harmondsworth: Penguin Books.

Asaad,G. and Shapiro,B. (1986) Hallucinations: Theoretical and Clinical Overview. *American Journal of Psychiatry*, 143:9.

Assagioli,R. (1975) *Psychosynthesis: A Manual of Principles and Techniques.* Wellingborough, Northamptonshire: Turnstone Press.

Aumann,J. (1967) Locutions. Catholic University of America (eds) *New Catholic Encyclopedia.* New York: McGraw-Hill.

Australian Broadcasting Commission (1984) *Barriers of the Mind* (Television Programme).

Barrett,T. and Etheridge,J. (1992) Verbal Hallucinations, I: People Who Hear 'Voices'. *Applied Cognitive Psychology*, Vol.6.

Barrett,W. (1986) *Death-Bed Visions.* Wellingborough, England: Aquarian Press.

Bateson,G. (ed) *Perceval's Narrative: A Patient's Account of His Psychosis.* California: Stanford University Press.

Beck,J. and Van der Kolk,B. (1987) Reports of Childhood Incest and Current Behaviour of Chronically Hospitalised Psychotic Women. *American Journal of Psychiatry*, 144:11.

Beckman,H. and Haas,S. (1980) High Dose Diazepam in Schizophrenia. *Psychopharmacology*, Vol.71.

Benjamin,L. (1989) Is Chronicity a Function of the Relationship Between the Person and the Auditory Hallucination? *Schizophrenia Bulletin*, Vol.15, No.2.

Bentall,R. (ed) (1990) *Reconstructing Schizophrenia*. London: Routledge.

Bentall,R., Jackson,H. and Pilgrim,D. (1988) Abandoning the Concept of 'Schizophrenia': Some Implications of Validity Arguments for Psychological Research into Psychotic Phenomena. *British Journal of Clinical Psychology*, Vol.27.

Bentall,R. and Slade,P. (1985) Reliability of a Measure of Disposition Towards Hallucination. *Personality and Individual Differences*, Vol.6.

Berne,E. (1975) *What Do You Say After You Say Hello?* London: Corgi Books.

Bilu,Y. and Abramovitch,H. (1985) In Search of the Saddiq: Visitational Dreams Among Moroccan Jews in Israel. *Psychiatry*, Vol.48.

Bleuler,E. (1950) *Dementia Praecox or the Group of Schizophrenias*. New York: International Universities Press.

Bleuler,M. (1979) On Schizophrenic Psychoses. *American Journal of Psychiatry*, 136:11.

Bliss,E. (1980) Multiple Personalities: A Report of 14 Cases with Implications for Schizophrenia and Hysteria. *Archives of General Psychiatry*, Vol.37.

Bliss,E., Larson,E. and Nakashima,S. (1983) Auditory Hallucinations and Schizophrenia. *Journal of Nervous and Mental Disease*, Vol.171, No.1.

Boisen,A. (1960) *Out of the Depths*. New York: Harper and Row.

Boisen,A. (1971) *The Exploration of the Inner World*. Philadelphia: University of Philadelphia Press.

Boon,S. and Draijer,N. (1993) Multiple Personality in the Netherlands: A Clinical Investigation of 71 Patients. *American Journal of Psychiatry*, 150:3.

Boss,M. (1963) *Psychoanalysis and Daseinanalysis*. New York: Basic Books.

Bourgignon,E. (1970) Hallucinations and Trance: An Anthropologist's Perspective. In Keup (ed.) *Origin and Mechanisms of Hallucinations*. New York: Plenum Press.

Boyle,M. (1993) *Schizophrenia: A Scientific Delusion?* London: Routledge.

Bragdon,E. (1990) *The Call of Spiritual Emergency*. San Francisco: Harper and Row.

Brauschi,J. and West,L. (1959) Sleep Deprivation. *Journal of the American Medical Association*, Vol.171.

Brier,A. and Strauss,J. (1983) Self-Control in Psychotic Disorders. *Archives of General Psychiatry*, Vol.40.

Brigitte, Sue, Mem and Veronika (1996) Power to Our Journeys. *American Family Therapy Academy Newsletter*, No.64.

Brown,R. (1971) *Unfinished Symphonies*. London: Souvenir Press.

Brown,R. (1975) *Immortals At My Elbow*. Melbourne: Hill of Content.

Bryer,J., Nelson,B., Miller,J. and Krol,P. (1987) Childhood Sexual and Physical Abuse as Factors in Adult Psychiatric Illness. *American Journal of Psychiatry*, 144: 11.

Bucke,R. (1961) *Cosmic Consciousness*. Secaucus, NJ: Citadel Press.

Carlson,G. and Goodwin,F. (1973) The Stages of Mania. *Archives of General Psychiatry*, Vol.28.

Carr,V. (1983) Recovery from Schizophrenia: A Review of Patterns of Psychosis. *Schizophrenia Bulletin*, Vol.9, No.1.

Carr,V. (1988) Patients' Techniques for Coping with Schizophrenia: An Exploratory Study. *British Journal of Medical Psychology*, Vol.61.

Casey,J. and Wilson,L. (1993) *The Flock*. London: Abacus.

Chadwick,P. and Birchwood,M. (1994) The Omnipotence of Voices: A Cognitive Approach to Auditory Hallucinations. *British Journal of Psychiatry*, Vol.164.

Chatterjee,M. (1984) *Gandhi's Religious Thought*. Notre Dame, IN: Notre Dame University Press.

Ciompi,L. (1984) Is There Really a Schizophrenia? The Long-Term Course of Psychotic Phenomena. *British Journal of Psychiatry*, Vol.145.

Clark,R. (1980) *Freud: The Man and the Cause*. London: Jonathan Cape.

Cleghorn,J., Franco,S., Szechtman,B., Kaplan,R., Szechtman,H., Brown,G., Nahmias,C. and Garnett,E. (1992) Toward a Brain Map of Auditory Hallucinations. *American Journal of Psychiatry*, 149:8.

Clifford,T. (1989) *The Diamond Healing: Tibetan Buddhist Medicine and Psychiatry*. Wellingborough, England: Aquarian Press.

Collins,M., Cull,C. and Sireling,L. (1989) Pilot Study of Treatment of Persistent Auditory Hallucinations by Modified Auditory Input. *British Medical Journal*, Vol.299.

Connell,J. (1992) *The Visions of the Children*. New York: St Martin's Press.

Corday,R. (1989) The Experience of Psychosis. *Journal of Contemplative Psychotherapy*, Vol.6.

Coté,I. (1994) Current Perspectives on Multiple Personality Disorder. *Hospital and Community Psychiatry*, Vol.45, No.8.

Craciunas,S. (1961) *The Lost Footsteps*. London: Collins and Harvill Press.

Cristiani,L. (1977) *St Joan of Arc*. Boston: Daughters of St Paul.

Critchley,E., Denmark,J., Warren,F. and Wilson,K. (1981) Hallucinatory Experiences of Prelingually Profoundly Deaf Schizophrenics. *British Journal of Psychiatry*, Vol.138.

Cromwell,R. and Snyder,C. (eds) (1993) *Schizophrenia: Origins, Processes, Treatment, and Outcome*. Oxford: Oxford University Press.

Cross,R. (1914) *Socrates: The Man and His Mission*. London: Methuen.

De Beauvoir,S. (1963) *Memoirs of a Dutiful Daughter*. Harmondsworth: Penguin Books.

Dean,S., Plyler,C. and Dean,M. (1980) Should Psychic Studies Be Included in Psychiatric Education? An Opinion Survey. *American Journal of Psychiatry*, 137: 10.

Densen-Gerber,J. (1986) The Occurrence of Stigmata in Multiple Personality/ Dissociative States. In Braun,B. (ed) *Dissociative Disorders: 1986*. Chicago: Rush University.

Devereux,G. (ed) (1970) *Psychoanalysis and the Occult*. New York: International Universities Press.

Ehrenwald,J. (1978) *The ESP Experience*. New York: Basic Books.

Eigen,M. (1993) *The Psychotic Core*. Northvale, NJ: Jason Aronson.

Eliade,M. (1989) *Shamanism: Archaic Technique of Ecstasy*. London: Arkana.

Elkin,A. (1977) *Aboriginal Men of High Degree*. St Lucia: University of Queensland Press.

Ellenberger,H. (1970) *The Discovery of the Unconscious*. New York: Basic Books.

Ensink,B. (1992) *Confusing Realities: A Study on Child Sexual Abuse and Psychiatric Symptoms*. Amsterdam: Free University Press.

Erickson,M. (1969) A Special Inquiry With Aldous Huxley Into the Nature and Character of Various States of Consciousness. In Tart,C. (ed.) *Altered States of Consciousness*. New York: Anchor Books.

Eshowsky,M. (1993) Practicing Shamanism in a Community Health Center. *Shamanism*, Vol.5, No.4 and Vol.6, No.1 (Double Issue)

Esquirol,J. (1965) Mental Maladies: A Treatise on Insanity (Facsimile of the English Edition of 1845). New York: Hafner.

Falloon,I. (1987) Cognitive and Behavioural Interventions in the Self Control of Schizophrenia. In Strauss,J., Böker,W. and Brenner,H. (eds) *Psychosocial Treatment of Schizophrenia*. New York: Hans Huber.

Falloon,I. And Talbot,R. (1981) Persistent Auditory Hallucinations: Coping Mechanisms and Implications for Management. *Psychological Medicine*, Vol.11.

Farley,J., Woodruff,R. and Guze,S. (1968) The Prevalence of Hysteria and Conversion Symptoms. *British Journal of Psychiatry*, Vol.114.

Farr,E. (1982) A Personal Account of Schizophrenia. In Tsuang,M. *Schizophrenia: The Facts*. Oxford: Oxford University Press.

Feder,R. (1982) Auditory Hallucinations Treated by Radio Headphones. *American Journal of Psychiatry*, Vol.139.

Ferrucci,P. (1982) *What We May Be*. Wellingborough, Northamptonshire: Turnstone Press.

Field,W. (1985) Hearing Voices. *Journal of Psychosocial Nursing*, Vol.23, No.1.

Folkard,L. (1992) *The Rock Pillow*. South Fremantle, WA: Fremantle Arts Centre Press.

Forrer,G. (1960) Benign Auditory and Visual Hallucinations. *Archives of General Psychiatry*, Vol.3.

Foundation for Inner Peace (1985) *A Course in Miracles*. London: Arkana.

Fox,M. and Sheldrake,R. (1996) *The Physics of Angels*. San Francisco: HarperCollins.

Freud,S. (1966) *The Psychopathology of Everyday Life*. London: Ernest Benn.

Frith,C. (1979) Consciousness, Information Processing, and Schizophrenia. *British Journal of Psychiatry*, Vol.134.

Gabbard,G. (1992) Psychodynamic Psychiatry in the 'Decade of the Brain'. *American Journal of Psychiatry*, 149:8.

Galton,F. (1973) *Inquiries into Human Faculty and its Development*. New York: AMS Press.

Goetz,C., Tanner,C. and Klawans,H. (1982) Pharmacology of Hallucinations Induced by Long-Term Drug Therapy. *American Journal of Psychiatry*, 139:4.

Goff,D., Henderson,D. and Amico,E. (1992) Cigarette Smoking in Schizophrenia: Relationship to Psychopathology and Medication Side Effects. *American Journal of Psychiatry*, Vol.149, No.9.

Gould,L. (1950) Verbal Hallucinations as Automatic Speech: The Reactivation of Dormant Speech Habit. *American Journal of Psychiatry*, Vol.107.

Grassian,G. (1983) Psychopathology of Solitary Confinement. *American Journal of Psychiatry*, Vol.140.

Green,M. and Kinsbourne,M. (1990) Subvocal Activity and Auditory Hallucinations: Clues for Behavioural Treatments? *Schizophrenia Bulletin*, Vol.16, No.4.

Greene,R. (1978) Auditory Hallucination Reduction: First Person Singular. *Journal of Contemporary Psychotherapy*, Vol.9, No.2.

Greyson,B. (1977) Telepathy in Mental Illness: Deluge or Delusion? *Journal of Nervous and Mental Disease*, Vol.165, No.3.

Greyson,B. and Stevenson,I. (1980) The Phenomenology of Near Death Experiences. *American Journal of Psychiatry*, Vol.137.

Grimby,A. (1993) Bereavement Among Elderly People: Grief Reactions, Post-Bereavement Hallucinations and Quality of Life. *Acta Psychiatrica Scandinavica*, Vol.87.

Grof,S. (1985) *Beyond the Brain*. New York: State University of New York Press.

Grof,S. and Grof,C. (1990) *The Stormy Search for the Self*. Los Angeles: Jeremy Tarcher.

Guirdham,A. (1982) *The Psychic Dimensions of Mental Health*. Wellingborough, Northamptonshire: Turnstone Press.

Gurney,E., Myers,F. and Podmore,F. (1970) *Phantasms of the Living* (two volumes, originally published 1886). Gainesville, Florida: Scholars' Facsimiles and Reprints.

Haddock,G., Bentall,R. and Slade,P. (1996) Psychological Treatment of Auditory Hallucinations: Focusing or Distraction? In Haddock,G. and Slade,P. (eds)

Cognitive-Behavioural Interventions with Psychotic Disorders. London: Routledge.

Haddock,G. and Slade,P. (eds) (1996) *Cognitive-Behavioural Interventions with Psychotic Disorders*. London: Routledge.

Hall,R., Popkin,M. and Faillace,L. (1978) Physical Illness Presenting as a Psychiatric Disease. *Archives of General Psychiatry*, Vol.35.

Hamilton,J. (1985) Auditory Hallucinations in Nonverbal Quadriplegics. *Psychiatry*, Vol.48.

Hamilton,M. (ed) (1976) *Fish's Schizophrenia (Second Edition)*. Bristol: John Wright and Sons.

Hammeke,T., McQuillen,M. and Cohen,B. (1983) Musical Hallucinations Associated with Acquired Deafness. *Journal of Neurology, Neurosurgery and Psychiatry*, Vol.46.

Handel,M. (1987) *Unpublished Personal Account of Schizophrenia*.

Hardy,A. (1979) *The Spiritual Nature of Man: A Study of Contemporary Religious Experience*. Oxford: Clarendon Press.

Harner,M. (ed) (1973) *Hallucinogens and Shamanism*. New York: Oxford University Press.

Hatfield,A. and Lefley,H. (1993) *Surviving Mental Illness*. New York: Guildford Press.

Hay,D. (1982) *Exploring Inner Space*. Harmondsworth: Penguin Books.

Healy,D. (1989) Neuroleptics and Psychic Indifference: A Review. *Journal of the Royal Society of Medicine*, Vol.82.

Healy,D. (1990) *The Suspended Revolution: Psychiatry and Psychotherapy Re-examined*. London: Faber and Faber.

Healy,D. (1993) *Psychiatric Drugs Explained*. London: Mosby.

Heery,M. (1989) Inner Voice Experiences: An Exploratory Study of Thirty Cases. *Journal of Transpersonal Psychology*, Vol.21, No.1.

Hellerstein,D., Frosch,W. and Koenigsberg,H. (1987) The Clinical Significance of Command Hallucinations. *American Journal of Psychiatry*, 144:2.

Hillman,J. and Ventura,M. (1992) *We've Had a Hundred Years of Psychotherapy – And the World's Getting Worse*. San Francisco: HarperCollins.

Hoffman,R. (1986) Verbal Hallucinations and Language Production Processes in Schizophrenia. *Behavioural and Brain Sciences*, Vol.9.

Honig,A. (1973) *The Awakening Nightmare*. New York: Delta Books.

James,W. (1902) *The Varieties of Religious Experience*. New York: Random House.

James,W. (1948) *Psychology*. Cleveland: World Publishing Company.

James,W. (1986) *Essays in Psychical Research*. Harvard, MA: Harvard University Press.

Jaspers,K. (1963) *General Psychopathology*. Chicago: University of Chicago Press.

Jaynes,J. (1982) *The Origin of Consciousness in the Breakdown of the Bicameral Mind*. Boston: Houghton Mifflin.

Jaynes,J. (1986) Hearing Voices and the Bicameral Mind. In Hoffman,R. (1986) Verbal Hallucinations and Language Production Processes in Schizophrenia. *Behavioural and Brain Sciences*, Vol.9.

Johnson,R. (1989) *Inner Work*. San Francisco: Harper and Row.

Judkins,M. and Slade,P. (1981) A Questionnaire Study of Hostility in Persistent Auditory Hallucinations. *British Journal of Medical Psychology*, Vol.54.

Julian,R. (1987) Spiritual Discernment in Psychiatric Patients. *Journal of Religion and Health*, Vol.26, No.2.

Jung,C. (1937) Psychological Factors Determining Human Behaviour. In Read,H., Fordham,M. and Adler,G. (eds) *The Collected Works of C.G.Jung, Volume Eight: The Structure and Dynamics of the Psyche*. Princeton: Princeton University Press.

Jung,C. (1967) *Memories, Dreams, Reflections*. London: Fontana.

Jung,C. (1969) *On the Nature of the Psyche*. Princeton: Princeton University Press.

Jung,C. (1973) *C.G.Jung: Letters, Volume 2: 1951–1961*. Adler,G. (ed.) Princeton: Princeton University Press.

Jung,C. (1974) *The Psychology of Dementia Praecox*. New Jersey: Princeton University Press.

Jung,C. (1977) *Psychology and the Occult*. Princeton: Princeton University Press.

Junginger,J. (1990) Predicting Compliance with Command Hallucinations. *American Journal of Psychiatry*, 147:2.

Kalweit,H. (1988) *Dreamtime and Inner Space: The World of the Shaman*. Boston: Shambala.

Kanas,N. and Barr,M. (1984) Self-Control of Psychotic Productions in Schizophrenics (Letter). *Archives of General Psychiatry*, Vol.41.

Kaplan,B. (ed.) (1964) *The Inner World of Mental Illness*. New York: Harper and Row.

Kaplan,H. and Sadock,B. (1981) *Modern Synopsis of Comprehensive Textbook of Psychiatry/III (Third Edition)*. Baltimore: Williams and Wilkins.

Kaplan,H. and Sadock,B. (eds) (1989) *Comprehensive Textbook of Psychiatry (Fifth Edition)*. Baltimore: Williams and Wilkins.

Kelsey,M. (1978) *Discernment*. New York: Paulist Press.

Keshavan,M., David,A., Steingard,S. and Lishman,W. (1992) Musical Hallucinations: A Review and Synthesis. *Neuropsychiatry, Neuropsychology, and Behavioral Neurology*, Vol.5, No.3.

King,L. (1956) *Criminal Complaints: A True Account*. Harvard: Ronald Press.

Kingdon,D. and Turkington,D. (1991) The Use of Cognitive Behaviour Therapy with a Normalising Rationale in Schizophrenia. *Journal of Nervous and Mental Disease*, Vol.179.

Kluft,R. (1986) High Functioning Multiple Personality Patients. *Journal of Nervous and Mental Disease*, Vol.174.

Kroll,J. and Bachrach,B. (1982a) Medieval Visions and Contemporary Hallucinations. *Psychological Medicine*, Vol.12.

Kroll,J. and Bachrach,B. (1982b) Visions and Psychopathology in the Middle Ages. *Journal of Nervous and Mental Disease*, Vol.170, No.1.

Kulkarni,J., Copolov,D. and Keks,N. (1991) Biological Investigations. In Kosky,R., Eshkevari,H. and Carr,V. (eds) *Mental Health and Illness*. Sydney: Butterworth-Heinemann.

Lally,S. (1989) 'Does Being In Here Mean There Is Something Wrong With Me?' *Schizophrenia Bulletin*, Vol.15, No.2.

Larkin,A. (1979) The Form and Content of Schizophrenic Hallucinations. *American Journal of Psychiatry*, 136:7.

Leete,E. (1993) The Interpersonal Environment – A Consumer's Personal Recollection. In Hatfield,A. and Lefley,H. (1993) *Surviving Mental Illness*. New York: Guildford Press.

Leff,J. (1968) Perceptual Phenomena and Personality in Sensory Deprivation. *British Journal of Psychiatry*, Vol.114.

Levinson,H. (1966) Auditory Hallucinations in a Case of Hysteria. *British Journal of Psychiatry*, Vol.112.

Lewinsohn,P. (1968) Characteristics of Patients with Hallucinations. *Journal of Clinical Psychology*, Vol.24.

Liester,M. (1996) Inner Voices: Distinguishing Transcendent and Pathological Characteristics. *Journal of Transpersonal Psychology*, Vol.28, No.1.

Lilly,J. (1956) Mental Effects of Reduction of Ordinary Levels of Physical Stimuli on Intact, Healthy Persons. *Psychiatric Research Reports 5, American Psychiatric Association*.

Lindbergh,C. (1953) *The Spirit of St Louis*. New York: Charles Scribner's.

Lingjaerde,O. (1982) Effect of the Benzodiazepine Derivative Estazolam in Patients with Auditory Hallucinations: A Multicentre Double-Blind, Cross-Over Study. *Acta Psychiatrica Scandinavica*, Vol.65.

Lockhart,R. (1975) Mary's Dog is an Ear Mother: Listening to the Voices of Psychosis. *Psychological Perspectives*, Vol.6.

Lovejoy,M. (1984) Recovery from Schizophrenia: A Personal Odyssey. *Hospital and Community Psychiatry*, Vol.35, No.8.

Lukoff,D. (1985) The Diagnosis of Mystical Experiences with Psychotic Features. *Journal of Transpersonal Psychology*, Vol.17, No.2.

Lukoff,D. (1990) Divine Madness: Shamanistic Initiatory Crisis and Psychosis. *Shaman's Drum*, Winter, 1990–91.

MacDonald,N. (1960) Living With Schizophrenia. *Canadian Medical Association Journal*, Vol.82.

Macnab,F. (1966) *Estrangement and Relationship*. Bloomington: Indiana University Press.

Maitland,S. (1997) Whisper Who Dares. *Open Mind*, Vol.84.

304   *Hearing Voices*

Malinak,D., Hoyt,M. and Patterson,V. (1979) Adults' Reactions to the Death of a Parent: A Preliminary Study. *American Journal of Psychiatry*, 136:9.

Margo,A., Hemsley,D. and Slade,P. (1981) The Effects of Varying Auditory Input on Schizophrenic Hallucinations. *British Journal of Psychiatry*, Vol.139.

Masters,R. and Houston,J. (1966) *The Varieties of Psychedelic Experience*. New York: Dell Publishing Company.

Matchett, W. (1972) Repeated Hallucinatory Experiences as a Part of the Mourning Process Among Hopi Indian Women. *Psychiatry*, Vol.35.

Mavromatis,A. (1987) *Hypnagogia: The Unique State of Consciousness Between Wakefulness and Sleep*. New York: Routledge and Kegan Paul.

Mayer-Gross,W., Slater,E. and Roth,M. (1960) *Clinical Psychiatry* (Second Edition). London: Cassell and Company.

McGorry,P., Chanen,A., McCarthy,E., Van Riel,R., McKenzie,D. and Singh,B. (1991) Posttraumatic Stress Disorder Following Recent-Onset Psychosis. *Journal of Nervous and Mental Disease*, Vol.179, No.5.

McInnis,M. and Marks,I. (1990) Audiotape Therapy for Persistent Auditory Hallucinations. *British Journal of Psychiatry*, Vol.157.

McKellar,P. (1968) *Experience and Behaviour*. Harmondsworth: Penguin Books.

McKenna,B. and Libersat,H. (1987) *Miracles Do Happen*. London: Pan Books.

Meier,C. (1989) *Healing Dream and Ritual*. Einseideln: Daimon Verlag.

Michaux,H. (1974) *The Major Ordeals of the Mind*. London: Secker and Warburg.

Miller,L., O'Connor,E. and DiPasquale,T. (1993) Patients' Attitudes Toward Hallucinations. *American Journal of Psychiatry*, 150:4.

Milner,D. (ed) (1978) *Explorations of Consciousness*. Suffolk: Neville Spearman.

Modell,A. (1960) An Approach to the Nature of Auditory Hallucinations in Schizophrenia. *Archives of General Psychiatry*, Vol.3.

Moody,R. (1975) *Life After Life*. Atlanta, GA: Mockingbird Books.

Mott,R., Small,I. and Anderson,J. (1965) Comparative Study of Hallucinations. *Archives of General Psychiatry*, Vol.12.

Mueser,K. and Butler,R. (1987) Auditory Hallucinations in Combat-Related Chronic Posttraumatic Stress Disorder. *American Journal of Psychiatry*, 144:3.

Neihardt,J. (1988) *Black Elk Speaks: Being the Life Story of a Holy Man of the Oglala Sioux*. Lincoln, Nebraska: University of Nebraska Press.

Nelson,H., Thrasher,S. and Barnes,T. (1991) Practical Ways of Alleviating Auditory Hallucinations. *British Medical Journal*, Vol.302.

Nelson,J. (1990) *Healing the Split*. Los Angeles: Jeremy Tarcher.

Nelson,P. (1989) A Survey of Mystical, Visionary and Remote Perception Experiences. In Zollschan,G., Schumaker,J. and Walsh,G. (eds) *Exploring the Paranormal: Perspectives on Belief and Experience*. Lindfield, NSW: Unity Press.

Noll,R. (1987) The Presence of Spirits in Magic and Madness. In Nicholson,S. (ed)

Shamanism: An Expanded View of Reality. Wheaton, Ill.: The Theosophical Publishing House.

Noll,R. (1989) Multiple Personality, Dissociation, and C.G.Jung's Complex Theory. *Journal of Analytical Psychology,* Vol.34.

North,C. (1989) *Welcome, Silence.* New York: Avon Books.

Olson,P., Suddeth,J., Peterson,P. and Egelhoff,C. (1985) Hallucinations of Widowhood. *Journal of the American Geriatric Society,* Vol.33.

Osis,K. (1961) *Deathbed Observations by Physicians and Nurses.* Parapsychological Monographs No.3. New York: Parapsychology Foundation.

Osis,K. and Haraldsson,E. (1977) *At the Hour of Death.* New York: Avon.

Peck,M. (1985) *The Road Less Travelled.* London: Rider.

Penfield,W. (1976) *The Mystery of the Mind.* Princeton: Princeton University Press.

Perry,J. (1989) *The Far Side of Madness.* Dallas, Texas: Spring Publications.

Peterson,D. (ed) (1982) *A Mad People's History of Madness.* Pittsburgh: University of Pittsburgh Press.

Pitts,F., Winokur,G. and Stewart,M. (1961) Psychiatric Syndromes, Anxiety Symptoms and Responses to Stress in Medical Students. *American Journal of Psychiatry,* Vol.118.

Podvoll,E. (1990) *The Seduction of Madness.* New York: HarperCollins.

Porter,R. (1989) *A Social History of Madness.* New York: Dutton.

Posey,T. and Losch,M. (1983) Auditory Hallucinations of Hearing Voices in 375 Normal Subjects. *Imagination, Cognition and Personality,* Vol.3, No.2.

Rack,P. (1982) *Race, Culture and Mental Disorder.* London: Tavistock Publications.

Rees,W. (1971) The Hallucinations of Widowhood. *British Medical Journal,* 4:37–41.

Ribi,A. (1990) *Demons of the Inner World.* Boston: Shambala.

Richards,D. (1990) Dissociation and Transformation. *Journal of Humanistic Psychology,* Vol.30, No.3.

Rilke,R. (1954) *Letters to a Young Poet.* New York: W.W.Norton.

Rojcewicz,S. and Rojcewicz,R. (1997) The 'Human' Voices in Hallucinations. *Journal of Phenomenological Psychology,* Vol.28, No.1.

Rollin,H. (ed) (1980) *Coping With Schizophrenia.* London: National Schizophrenia Fellowship.

Romme,M. and Escher,A. (1989) Hearing Voices. *Schizophrenia Bulletin,* Vol.15, No.2.

Romme,M. and Escher,A. (1996) Empowering People Who Hear Voices. In Haddock,G. and Slade,P. (eds) *Cognitive-Behavioural Interventions with Psychotic Disorders.* London: Routledge.

Romme,M., Honig,A., Noorthoorn,E. and Escher,A. (1992) Coping with Hearing Voices: An Emancipatory Approach. *British Journal of Psychiatry,* Vol.161.

Rosenbaum,M. (1980) The Role of the Term Schizophrenia in the Decline of Diagnoses of Multiple Personality. *Archives of General Psychiatry*, Vol.37.

Rosenhan,D. (1973) On Being Sane in Insane Places. *Science*, Vol.179.

Ross,C. (1989) *Multiple Personality Disorder: Diagnosis, Clinical Features, and Treatment.* New York: John Wiley and Sons.

Ross,C., Miller,S., Reagor,P., Bjornson,L., Fraser,G. and Anderson,G. (1990) Schneiderian Symptoms in Multiple Personality Disorder and Schizophrenia. *Comprehensive Psychiatry*, Vol.31, No.2.

Rowan,J. (1993) *Discover Your Subpersonalities.* London: Routledge.

Ryan,L. and Ross,C. (1988) Dissociation in Adolescents and College Students. In Braun,B. (ed) *Dissociative Disorders: 1988.* Chicago: Rush University.

Sabom,M. (1982) *Recollections of Death.* New York: Harper and Row.

Sacks,O. (1991) *Awakenings.* London: Pan Books.

Sandford,J. and Sandford,P. (1985) *Healing the Wounded Spirit.* Tulsa, OK: Victory House.

Sanford,J. (1977) *Healing and Wholeness.* New York: Paulist Press.

Sarbin,T. and Juhasz,J. (1967) The Historical Background of the Concept of Hallucination. *Journal of the History of the Behavioural Sciences*, Vol.3.

Sartorius,N., Shapiro,R. and Jablensky,A. (1974) The International Pilot Study of Schizophrenia. *Schizophrenia Bulletin*, Vol.1.

Schatzberg,A. and Rothschild,A. (1992) Psychotic (Delusional) Major Depression. *American Journal of Psychiatry*, 149:6.

Schreber,D. (1955) *Memoirs of My Nervous Illness.* Edited and Translated by I.Macalpine and R.Hunter. London: William Dawson and Sons.

Schreiber,F. (1973) *Sybil.* Harmondsworth: Penguin Books.

Sechehaye,M. (ed) (1970) *Autobiography of a Schizophrenic Girl.* New York: New American Library.

Shaw,B. (1957) *St Joan.* London: Longmans Green and Company.

Sidgwick,H., Sidgwick,E. and Johnson,A. (1894) Report on the Census of Hallucinations. *Proceedings of the Society for Psychical Research*, Vol.10.

Siegel,R. (1984) Hostage Hallucinations. *Journal of Nervous and Mental Disease*, Vol.172.

Singer,J. (1973a) *The Child's World of Make Believe: Experimental Studies of Imaginative Play.* New York: Academic Press.

Singer,J. (1973b) *Boundaries of the Soul.* New York: Anchor Books.

Sirota,P., Spivac,B. and Meshulam,B. (1987) Conversive Hallucinations. *British Journal of Psychiatry*, Vol.151.

Sizemore,C. and Pittillo,E. (1978) *Eve.* London: Victor Gollancz.

Slade,P. (1976) Towards a Theory of Auditory Hallucinations: Outline of an Hypothetical Four-Factor Model. *British Journal of Social and Clinical Psychology*, Vol.15.

Slade,P. (1990) The Behavioural and Cognitive Treatment of Psychotic Symptoms. In Bentall,R. (ed) (1990) *Reconstructing Schizophrenia*. London: Routledge.

Slade,P. and Bentall,R. (1988) *Sensory Deception: A Scientific Analysis of Hallucination*. Baltimore: The Johns Hopkins University Press.

Slocum,J. (1978) *Sailing Alone Around the World*. London: Granada.

Smith,F. (1997) *Personal Communication*.

Smith,J. (1992) The Auditory Hallucinations of Schizophrenia. In Reisberg,D. (ed) *Auditory Imagery*. Hillsdale, NJ: Lawrence Erlbaum.

St John of the Cross (1964) The Ascent of Mount Carmel. In *The Collected Works of St John of the Cross* (Translated by Kavanaugh,K. and Rodriguez,O.). London: Nelson.

Starbuck,E. (1899) *The Psychology of Religion*. London: Walter Scott.

Stephen,M. (1989) Self, the Sacred Other, and Autonomous Imagination. In Herdt,G. and Stephen,M. (eds) *The Religious Imagination in New Guinea*. London: Rutgers University Press.

Stevenson,I. (1983) Do We Need a New Word to Supplement 'Hallucination'? *American Journal of Psychiatry*, 140:12.

Stokes,D. and Dearsley,L. (1980) *Voices in My Ear – The Autobiography of a Medium*. London: Futura Publications.

Stone,H. and Winkelman,S. (1989) *Embracing Our Selves*. San Rafael, California: New World Library.

Storr,A. (1983) (ed.) *Jung: Selected Writings*. London: Fontana.

Storr,A. (1989) *Solitude: A Return to the Self*. New York: Ballantine.

Strauss,J. (1969) Hallucinations and Delusions as Points on Continua Function. *Archives of General Psychiatry*, Vol.21.

Strauss,J. (1989) Subjective Experience of Schizophrenia: Toward a New Dynamic Psychiatry II. *Schizophrenia Bulletin*, Vol.15, No.2.

Sutherland,C. (1993) *Within the Light*. Sydney: Bantam Books.

Swedenborg,E. (1971) *Heaven and Hell*. New York: Swedenborg Foundation.

Talmage,J. (1970) *Jesus the Christ*. Salt Lake City, Utah: Deseret Book Company.

Tarrier,N. (1992) Management and Modification of Residual Positive Psychotic Symptoms. In Birchwood,C. and Tarrier,N. (eds) *Innovations in the Psychological Management of Schizophrenia*. New York: John Wiley and Sons.

Taylor,M. and Abrams,R. (1975) Acute Mania: Clinical and Genetic Study of Responders and Nonresponders to Treatments. *Archives of General Psychiatry*, Vol.32.

Teresa of Avila (1979) *The Interior Castle*. New York: Paulist Press.

Thigpen,C. and Cleckley,H. (1957) *The Three Faces of Eve*. New York: Secker and Warburg.

Thomas à Kempis (1963) *The Imitation of Christ*. London: Fontana.

Thomas,P. (1997) *The Dialectics of Schizophrenia*. London: Free Association Books.

Tien,A. (1991) Distributions of Hallucinations in the Population. *Social Psychiatry and Psychiatric Epidemiology*, Vol.26.

Tiihonen,J., Hari,R., Naukkarinen,H., Rimón,R., Jousmäki,V. and Kajola,M. (1992) Modified Activity of the Human Auditory Cortex During Auditory Hallucinations. *American Journal of Psychiatry*, 149:2.

Torrey,E. (1988) *Surviving Schizophrenia*. New York: Harper and Row.

Tyrrell,G. (1953) *Apparitions*. London: Gerald Duckworth.

Underhill,E. (1990) *Mysticism*. New York: Doubleday.

Van Dusen,W. (1972) *The Natural Depth in Man*. New York: Swedenborg Foundation.

Van Dusen,W. (1973) The Presence of Spirits in Madness. In Fadiman,J. and Kewman,D. (eds) *Exploring Madness: Experience, Theory, and Research*. California: Brooks Cole.

Vonnegut,M. (1976) *The Eden Express*. New York: Bantam Books.

Walsh,R. (1990) *The Spirit of Shamanism*. London: HarperCollins.

Warner,R. (1985) *Recovery From Schizophrenia*. London: Routledge and Kegan Paul.

Watkins,J. (1996) *Living With Schizophrenia*. Melbourne: Hill Of Content.

Watkins,M. (1990) *Invisible Guests: The Development of Imaginal Dialogues*. Boston: Sigo Press.

Weingaertner,A. (1971) Self-Administered Aversive Stimulation with Hallucinating Hospitalised Schizophrenics. *Journal of Consulting and Clinical Psychology*, Vol.36, No.3.

West,D. (1948) A Mass Observation Questionnaire on Hallucinations. *Journal of the Society for Psychical Research*, Vol.34.

Whitwell,F. and Barker,M. (1980) 'Possession' in Psychiatric Patients in Britain. *British Journal of Medical Psychology*, Vol.53.

Wilcox,J., Briones,D. and Suess,L. (1991) Auditory Hallucinations, Posttraumatic Stress Disorder, and Ethnicity. *Comprehensive Psychiatry*, Vol.32, No.4.

Will,O. (1962) Hallucinations: Comments Reflecting Clinical Observations of the Schizophrenic Reaction. In West,L. (ed.) *Hallucinations*. New York: Grune and Stratton.

Wing,J. (1978) *Reasoning About Madness*. Oxford: Oxford University Press.

Yamamoto,J., Okonogi,K., Iwasaki,T. and Yosimura,S. (1969) Mourning in Japan. *American Journal of Psychiatry*, Vol.125.

Young,H., Bentall,R., Slade,P. and Dewey,M. (1986) Disposition Toward Hallucination, Gender and IQ Scores. *Personality and Individual Differences*, Vol.7.

Zuckerman,M. (1969) Variables Affecting Deprivation Results. In Zubek,J. (ed) *Sensory Deprivation: Fifteen Years of Research*. New York: Appleton-Century-Crofts.

Zollschan,G., Schumaker,J. and Walsh,G. (eds) *Exploring the Paranormal: Perspectives on Belief and Experience*. Lindfield, NSW: Unity Press.

INDEX

First published 1998
This new edition published 2008
Reprinted 2013
by Michelle Anderson Publishing Pty Ltd
P O Box 6032
Chapel Street North
South Yarra 3141
www.michelleandersonpublishing.com
mapubl@bigpond.net.au

© Copyright: John Watkins 2008

Cover design: Naro street corporate communications
Typeset by: Midland Typesetters, Maryborough, Australia
Printed by: Toppan Security Printing Pte. Ltd.

National Library of Australia cataloguing-in-publication entry

Watkins, John, 1951-

Hearing voices : a common human experience / John Watkins

Rev. ed.

Melbourne, Vic. : Michelle Anderson Publishing, 2008.

l v.

ISBN 9780855723903 (pbk.)

Includes index.
Bibliography.

Hallucinations and illusions.
Mental illness – Treatment.
Schizophrenia – Treatment.

152.15